HANDBOOK OF COMMON ORTHOPAEDIC FRACTURES AND DRUGS

First Edition

Scott Hal Kozin, M.D.
Assistant Professor of Orthopaedic Surgery
Temple University School of Medicine
Philadelphia, Pennsylvania

Anthony Clayton Berlet, M.D.
Assistant Clinical Professor
Department of Plastic and Reconstructive Surgery
UMDNJ - New Jersey Medical School
Newark, New Jersey

2003

HANDBOOK OF COMMON ORTHOPAEDIC FRACTURES AND DRUGS

First Edition

 MSI

Illustrations by Anthony C. Berlet, M.D.

PREFACE

Orthopaedic surgery is a field of medicine that encompasses a wide spectrum of disease entities and fractures. Fractures may occur anywhere in the human and accurate assessment is essential for diagnosis and treatment. Fractures throughout the body have been extensively analyzed and classified. These classifications are based on fracture configurations, mechanism of injury or fracture stability. This has led to an overwhelming number of classifications and eponyms which are frequently confusing and cumbersome. In addition, many fractures have multiple classifications creating further confusion. A classification should provide therapeutic and prognostic information to be valuable in fracture management.

The First Edition of the **HANDBOOK OF COMMON ORTHOPAEDIC FRACTURES AND DRUGS** is published for the practicing physician, resident, medical student and other health care professionals to simplify fracture classifications, help access fracture stability, and direct treatment. All fractures should initially be described according to length, angulation, rotation, displacement, and degree of comminution, prior to attempting specific classification. These variables are essential in orthopaedic analysis for treatment of fractures and are incorporated in many of the classification schemas. This handbook contains the majority of fractures that have been appropriately classified and includes an Eponym section for reference purposes. Extremely uncommon fractures and those without adequate classification are not included in this text.

This handbook is organized into seven sections: (1) Upper Extremity, (2) Spine, (3) Pelvis and Acetabulum, (4) Lower Extremity, (5) Pediatrics, and (6) Osteonecrosis and Osteochondrosis and (7) Eponyms. The fracture classifications are listed in a distal to proximal direction for the Upper Extremity followed by a cephalad to caudad direction for the remaining sections. The Eponym section is listed in alphabetical order and includes adult and pediatric nomenclature. This organization is designed to allow quick and easy reference to specific fracture classifications.

Also included in this edition is a new section on various commonly used drugs in orthopaedics. The section includes information for the medical community with a concise reference source for drug names and the preparations available with common dosages in adults in a tabular format.

The **HANDBOOK OF COMMON ORTHOPAEDIC FRACTURES AND DRUGS, First Edition**, is physically designed to fit in a pocket to allow for easy accessibility. We hope this text will be useful in simplifying fracture assessment and classifications. We continue to welcome any suggestions, comments, and criticisms that may improve our handbook.

We wish to thank Edward J. Barbieri, Ph.D., and G. John DiGregorio, M.D., Ph.D., for their assistance with the composition and preparation of this handbook.

Scott H. Kozin, M.D.
Anthony C. Berlet, M.D.

TABLE OF CONTENTS

INTRODUCTION

Orthopaedic fracture management begins with initial patient evaluation. The entire patient and involved extremity should be carefully and thoroughly examined. A complete neurovascular examination of the potentially fractured extremity is vital in the initial assessment. Neurovascular compromise is an orthopaedic emergency and requires prompt therapeutic intervention. All fractures should be initially splinted to prevent further tissue damage and for patient comfort. The skin should be inspected for evidence of bone penetration leading to open fracture management. Open fractures require cultures, debridement, antibiotics, and sterile dressings as part of their initial management. Radiographic analysis should be prompt and should include the joint above and below the fracture; for example, a femoral shaft fracture should have radiographic visualization of the entire femur including the femoral head and condyles.

After careful history, physical examination, and radiography, an appropriate description of the fracture should be formulated. Orthopaedic fracture description is based upon length, angulation, rotation, and degree of bony comminution. A fractured extremity may be shortened or distracted, angulated in multiple directions, malrotated, or severely comminuted. All of these factors influence the therapeutic decision process and effect overall prognosis. Fractures should also be described as open with bone penetration of the skin or closed with preservation of the overlying skin. Fracture description should include the overlying soft tissue damage as well as the disruption of underlying bone and neurovascular elements. These variables all are indicative of the amount of energy absorbed by the fractured extremity at the time of injury. These factors are major determinants in the overall prognosis of the injured extremity.

Many fractures have been organized into classification schemas to provide therapeutic and prognostic information valuable in fracture management. This third edition text organizes those orthopaedic classifications into six expanded sections:

(1)   Upper Extremity,
(2)   Spine,
(3)   Pelvis and Acetabulum,
(4)   Lower Extremity, and
(5)   Pediatrics.
(6)   Osteonecrosis and Osteochondrosis

The Upper Extremity classifications are listed in a distal to proximal direction beginning with distal phalangeal fractures and progressing proximally including Frykman's classification of wrist fractures, Mason's classifications of radial head fractures, and Neer's classification of proximal humeral fractures. Each fracture classification is accompanied by extensive illustrations to aid in the understanding and application of specific classification schemas.

1

The Spine section progresses from a cephalad to caudad direction and includes cervical and thoracolumbar fractures. There is a separate section dedicated to odontoid fractures with illustrations in both the anteroposterior and lateral views.

The third section concentrates on pelvis and acetabular fractures. Tile's classification of pelvic disruption and acetabular fractures was selected because of its valuable therapeutic and prognostic information. This classification is presented in outline form with detailed illustrations to simplify its application in the clinical setting.

The fourth section involves the entire lower extremity beginning with hip fractures. These fractures are divided into femoral neck, intertrochanteric and subtrochanteric classifications. Accurate classification of these common fractures is necessary to select appropriate treatment. This section lists fractures in a superior to inferior direction and includes Winquist's classification of femoral shaft comminution, Hawkin's classification of talar neck fractures, and Essex-Lopresti's classification of calcaneus fractures. Ankle fractures are commonly classified according to either the Lauge-Hansen or Danis-Weber schema. Therefore, both of these classifications are included in this text.

The fifth section discusses pediatric fractures beginning with the Salter-Harris classification of physeal disruptions. This classification is used to describe the majority of pediatric fractures. Additional specific upper and lower extremity schemas are presented to complete this section.

The new sixth section concerns the topics osteonecrosis and osteochondrosis. The diagnosis of osteonecrosis indicates that the ischemic death of bone and marrow has occurred. The diagnosis of osteochondrosis initially was interpreted as primary impairment of local blood supply that led to a similar sequence as osteonecrosis. However, further investigation into osteochondrosis has determined that many cases of ostechondrosis do not have histologic evidence of dead bone. Therefore, these two entities overlap and are included in a single section that describes this heterogeneous group of disorders.

The seventh section of this handbook is dedicated to fracture eponyms. Eponyms to describe various fracture configurations are commonly employed. An alphabetical listing of fracture eponyms with illustrations and references is presented to allow easy accessibility.

The organization into these various sections is to allow an easily accessible reference text to specific fracture classifications and eponyms. The detailed illustrations are to simplify the understanding of these classification schemas. Hopefully, this combination of text and illustrations will simplify orthopaedic fracture classifications and be useful in the clinical setting.

UPPER EXTREMITY

DISTAL PHALANX FRACTURES

(Kaplan Classification)

I. LONGITUDINAL

II. TRANSVERSE

III. COMMINUTED

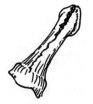

I. Longitudinal

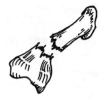

II. Transverse

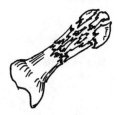

III. Comminuted

BASE OF THUMB METACARPAL FRACTURES

(Green Classification)

INTRA-ARTICULAR FRACTURES

    I.   BENNETT'S FRACTURE

    II.   ROLANDO'S FRACTURE

EXTRA-ARTICULAR FRACTURES

    III.   FRACTURES OF THE METACARPAL BASE

          A.   TRANSVERSE

          B.   OBLIQUE

    IV.   EPIPHYSEAL FRACTURE

6

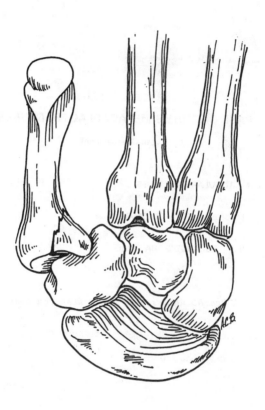

BASE OF THUMB METACARPAL FRACTURES

(Green Classification)

INTRA-ARTICULAR FRACTURES

    I.   BENNETT'S FRACTURE

    II.   ROLANDO'S FRACTURE

BENNETT'S and ROLANDO's FRACTURES are further described in the EPONYM SECTION.

I. Bennett's
Fracture

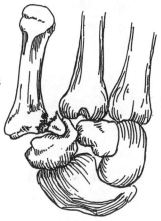

II. Rolando's
Fracture

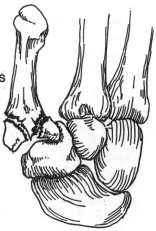

BASE OF THUMB METACARPAL FRACTURES

(Green Classification)

EXTRA-ARTICULAR FRACTURES

    III.   FRACTURES OF THE METACARPAL BASE

        A.   TRANSVERSE

        B.   OBLIQUE

    IV. EPIPHYSEAL FRACTURE

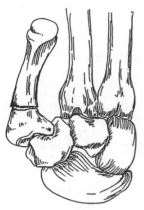

IIIA. Transverse

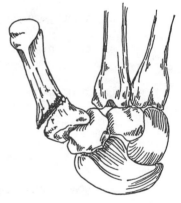

IIIB. Oblique

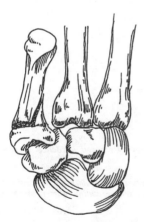

IV. Epiphyseal

SCAPHOID FRACTURES

(Russe Classification)

ANATOMIC LOCATION

    I.   PROXIMAL THIRD - 20%[a]

    II.   MIDDLE THIRD - 70%

    III. DISTAL THIRD - 10%

FRACTURE CONFIGURATION

    I.   TRANSVERSE

    II.   VERTICAL OBLIQUE

    III. HORIZONTAL OBLIQUE

Proximal third scaphoid fractures have increased incidence of avascular necrosis.

Forces across the wrist tend to compress and stabilize the horizontal oblique and transverse scaphoid fractures. The vertical oblique configuration tends to displace as the forces shear the fracture surface.

[a] *Percentages indicate the frequency of fracture occurrence.*

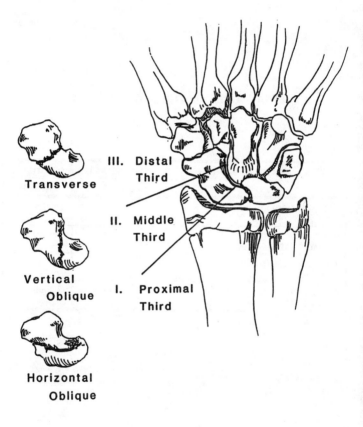

Transverse

Vertical Oblique

Horizontal Oblique

III. **Distal Third**

II. **Middle Third**

I. **Proximal Third**

FRACTURES OF THE DISTAL RADIUS

(Frykman Classification)

FRACTURE PATTERN	DISTAL ULNA FRACTURE	
	ABSENT	PRESENT
EXTRA-ARTICULAR	I	II
INTRA-ARTICULAR INVOLVING RADIOCARPAL JOINT	III	IV
INTRA-ARTICULAR INVOLVING RADIOULNAR JOINT	V	VI
INTRA-ARTICULAR INVOLVING RADIOCARPAL and RADIOULNAR JOINTS	VII	VIII

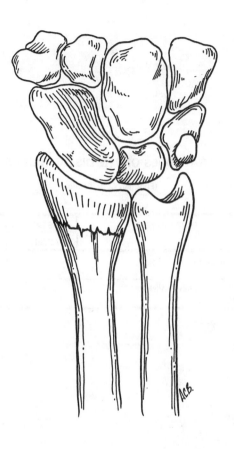

FRACTURES OF THE DISTAL RADIUS

(Frykman Classification)

FRACTURE PATTERN	DISTAL ULNA FRACTURE	
	ABSENT	PRESENT
EXTRA-ARTICULAR	I	II
INTRA-ARTICULAR INVOLVING RADIOCARPAL JOINT	III	IV

I.

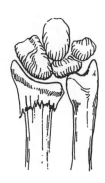

II.

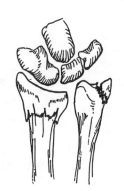

III.

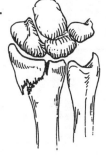

IV.

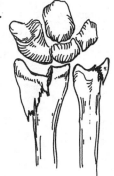

FRACTURES OF THE DISTAL RADIUS

(Frykman Classification)

FRACTURE PATTERN	DISTAL ULNA FRACTURE	
	ABSENT	PRESENT
INTRA-ARTICULAR INVOLVING RADIOULNAR JOINT	V	VI
INTRA-ARTICULAR INVOLVING RADIOCARPAL and RADIOULNAR JOINTS	VII	VIII

V.

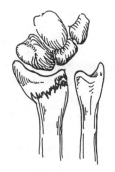

VI.

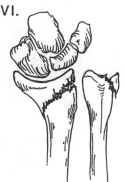

VII.

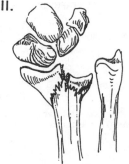

VIII.

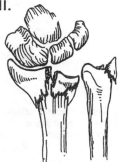

FRACTURES OF THE PROXIMAL ULNA
WITH RADIAL HEAD DISLOCATION - MONTEGGIA LESION

(Bado Classification)

I. ANTERIOR DISLOCATION OF THE RADIAL HEAD AND FRACTURE OF THE ULNAR DIAPHYSIS AT ANY LEVEL WITH ANTERIOR ANGULATION

II. POSTERIOR OR POSTEROLATERAL DISLOCATION OF THE RADIAL HEAD AND FRACTURE OF THE ULNAR DIAPHYSIS WITH POSTERIOR ANGULATION

III. LATERAL OR ANTEROLATERAL DISLOCATION OF THE RADIAL HEAD AND FRACTURE OF THE ULNAR METAPHYSIS

IV. ANTERIOR DISLOCATION OF THE RADIAL HEAD, FRACTURE OF THE THE PROXIMAL THIRD OF THE RADIUS, AND FRACTURE OF THE THE ULNA AT THE SAME LEVEL

Type I fracture dislocation is the most common type, accounting for approximately 65 percent of Monteggia lesions. Type IV lesions are uncommon, less than 5 percent of total.

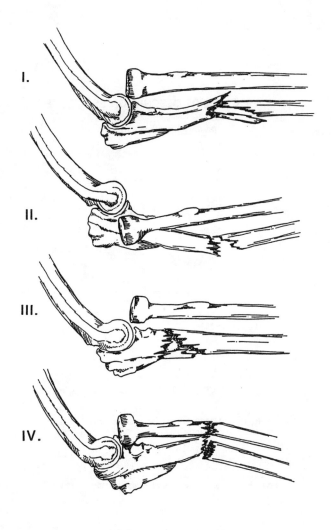

I.

II.

III.

IV.

CLASSIFICATION OF OLECRANON FRACTURES

(Morrey Classification)

I.   UNDISPLACED

    A.   NONCOMMINUTED

    B.   COMMINUTED

II.   DISPLACED - STABLE

    A.   NONCOMMINUTED

    B.   COMMINUTED

III.   DISPLACED - UNSTABLE

    A.   NONCOMMINUTED

    B.   COMMINUTED

The higher fracture types have less satisfactory results.

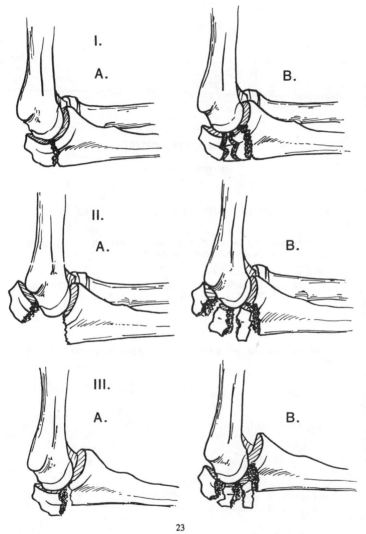

CORONOID FRACTURES

(Morrey Classification)

I.   AVULSION OF THE TIP OF THE CORONOID PROCESS

II.   SINGLE OR COMMINUTED FRAGMENT INVOLVING 50 PERCENT OR LESS OF THE CORONOID PROCESS

III.   SINGLE OR COMMINUTED FRAGMENT INVOLVING GREATER THAN 50 PERCENT OF THE CORONOID PROCESS

Coronoid fractures are uncommon and often associated with elbow dislocations.

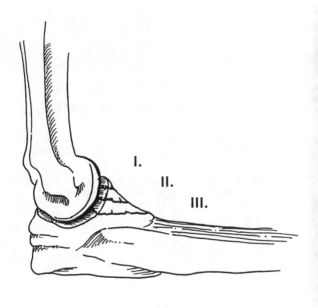

I.

II.

III.

FRACTURES OF THE RADIAL HEAD

(Mason Classification with Johnston Modification)

I. NONDISPLACED LINEAR OR TRANSVERSE FRACTURES - 50%[a]

II. FRACTURES WITH MINIMAL DISPLACEMENT OR COMMINUTED
    FRACTURES WITHOUT DISPLACEMENT - 20%

III. COMMINUTED FRACTURES WITH MARKED DISPLACEMENT - 20%

IV. RADIAL HEAD FRACTURES WITH ELBOW DISLOCATION - 10%

Most common elbow fracture in adults.

[a] *Percentages indicate the frequency of fracture occurrence.*

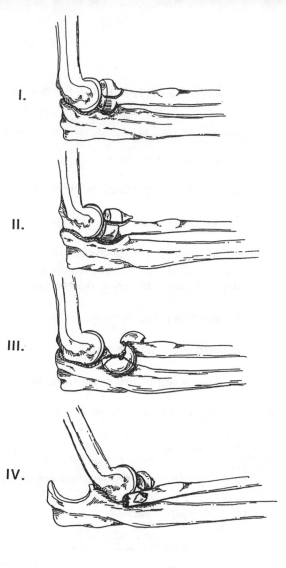

I.

II.

III.

IV.

FRACTURES OF THE DISTAL HUMERUS

(Muller Classification)

A. EXTRA-ARTICULAR FRACTURES

    A1. AVULSION FRACTURES OF THE EPICONDYLES

    A2. SIMPLE SUPRACONDYLAR FRACTURE

    A3. COMMINUTED SUPRACONDYLAR FRACTURE

B. INTRA-ARTICULAR FRACTURES OF ONE CONDYLE

    B1. FRACTURE OF THE TROCHLEA

    B2. FRACTURE OF THE CAPITELLUM

    B3. TANGENTIAL FRACTURE OF THE TROCHLEA

C. BI-CONDYLAR FRACTURES

    C1. Y-FRACTURE

    C2. Y-FRACTURE WITH SUPRACONDYLAR COMMINUTION

    C3. COMMINUTED FRACTURE

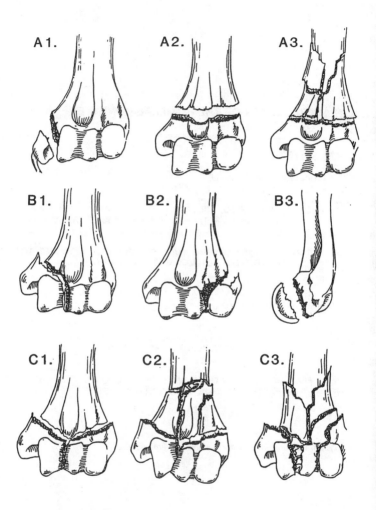

FRACTURES OF THE HUMERAL CONDYLES

(Milch Classification)

LATERAL HUMERAL CONDYLE

I.   SIMPLE FRACTURE OF THE LATERAL CONDYLE WITH LATERAL WALL OF TROCHLEA ATTACHED TO MAIN MASS OF THE HUMERUS

II.   FRACTURE WITH LATERAL WALL OF TROCHLEA ATTACHED TO FRACTURED LATERAL CONDYLAR FRAGMENT

MEDIAL LATERAL CONDYLE

I.   SIMPLE FRACTURE OF MEDIAL CONDYLE WITH LATERAL WALL OF TROCHLEA ATTACHED TO MAIN MASS OF THE HUMERUS

II.   FRACTURE WITH LATERAL WALL OF TROCHLEA ATTACHED TO FRACTURED MEDIAL CONDYLAR FRAGMENT

Type II fractures involve the trochlea and are unstable.

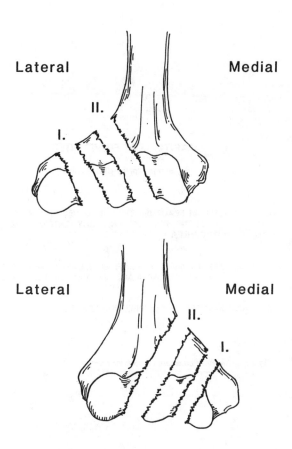

Lateral   Medial

Lateral   Medial

CAPITELLUM FRACTURES

(Bryan and Morrey Classification)

I. CAPITELLUM FRACTURE THAT INVOLVES THE MAJORITY OF THE OSSEOUS PORTION AND MAY EXTEND INTO ADJACENT TROCHLEA

II. SLICE FRACTURE OF THE CAPITELLUM WITH VARIABLE AMOUNT OF ARTICULAR CARTILAGE AND MINIMAL SUBCHONDRAL BONE

III. COMMINUTED OR COMPRESSION FRACTURE

Type I is the most common capitellum fracture.

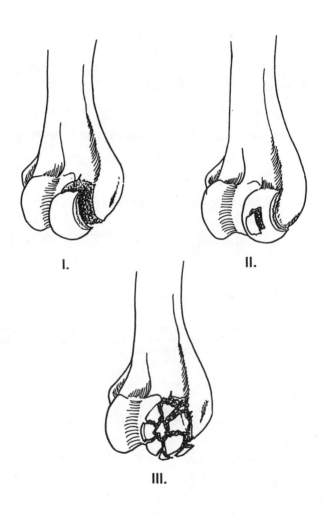

I.

II.

III.

INTERCONDYLAR FRACTURES OF THE HUMERUS

(Riseborough and Radin Classification)

I.   NO DISPLACEMENT OF THE FRAGMENTS

II.   T-SHAPED FRACTURE WITH THE TROCHLEAR AND CAPITELLAR FRAGMENTS SEPARATED BUT NOT APPRECIABLY ROTATED IN THE FRONTAL PLANE

III.   T-SHAPED FRACTURE WITH SEPARATION OF THE FRAGMENTS AND SIGNIFICANT ROTARY DEFORMITY

IV.   T-SHAPED INTERCONDYLAR FRACTURES WITH SEVERE COMMINUTION OF THE ARTICULAR SURFACE AND WIDE SEPARATION OF THE HUMERUS CONDYLES

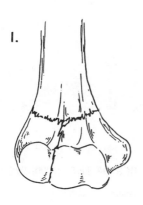

I.

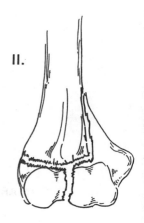

II.

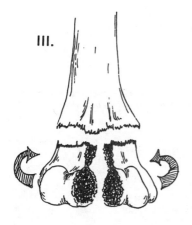

III.

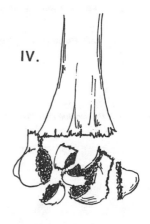

IV.

35

TRANSCONDYLAR FRACTURES OF THE HUMERUS

(Ashurst Classification)

I.   POSTERIOR DISPLACEMENT

II.   ANTERIOR DISPLACEMENT

TRANSCONDYLAR FRACTURES are intercapsular fractures through the condyles. Displacement of the dicondylar fragment is usually posterior.

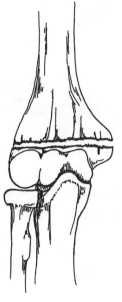

Transcondylar

I. Posterior

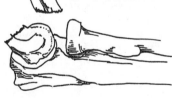

II. Anterior

SUPRACONDYLAR FRACTURES OF THE HUMERUS

(Modified Kocher Classification)

I. EXTENSION TYPE

II. FLEXION TYPE

SUPRACONDYLAR EXTENSION FRACTURES are more common than the FLEXION TYPE and approximately 50 percent are completely displaced.

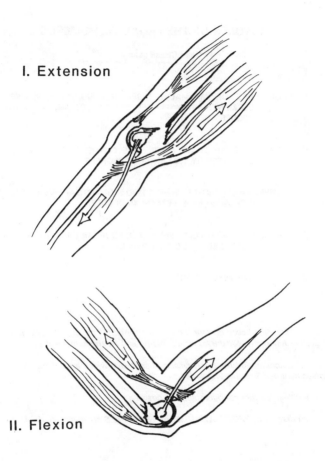

I. Extension

II. Flexion

FRACTURES OF THE PROXIMAL HUMERUS

(Neer Classification)

I.   ONE-PART OR MINIMALLY DISPLACED FRACTURE WHERE NO SEGMENTS ARE DISPLACED BY 1.0 CM OR ANGULATED BY 45 DEGREES

II. TWO-PART FRACTURE WHERE ONE SEGMENT IS SIGNIFICANTLY DISPLACED BY 1.0 CM OR 45 DEGREES

III. THREE-PART FRACTURE WHERE TWO SEGMENTS ARE SIGNIFICANTLY DISPLACED BY 1.0 CM OR 45 DEGREES

IV. FOUR-PART FRACTURE WHERE ALL FOUR MAJOR SEGMENTS ARE DISPLACED BY 1.0 CM OR 45 DEGREES

V.   FRACTURE DISLOCATION

Classification based on four fracture segments: (1) the articular segment, (2) the greater tuberosity, (3) the lesser tuberosity, and (4) the humeral shaft.

Classification describes only displaced segments which are defined as 1.0 cm displacement or 45 degree angulation.

Multiple fracture configurations are possible.

80 percent of PROXIMAL HUMERAL FRACTURES are minimally displaced.

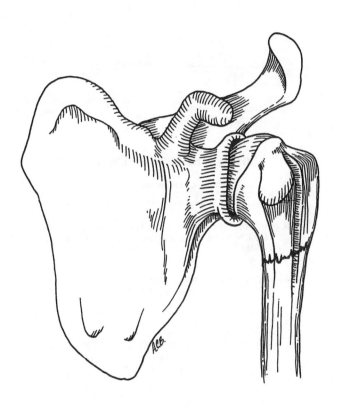

FRACTURES OF THE PROXIMAL HUMERUS

(Neer Classification)

I.   ONE-PART OR MINIMALLY DISPLACED FRACTURE WHERE NO SEGMENTS ARE DISPLACED BY 1.0 CM OR ANGULATED BY 45 DEGREES

II.   TWO-PART FRACTURE WHERE ONE SEGMENT IS SIGNIFICANTLY DISPLACED BY 1.0 CM OR 45 DEGREES

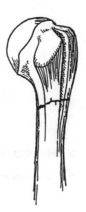

One Part Fracture

Two Part

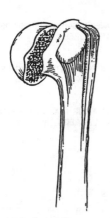

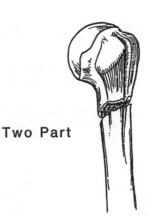

Articular Segment
Fracture

Humeral Shaft
Fracture

FRACTURES OF THE PROXIMAL HUMERUS

(Neer Classification)

I. ONE-PART OR MINIMALLY DISPLACED FRACTURE WHERE NO SEGMENTS ARE DISPLACED BY 1.0 CM OR ANGULATED BY 45 DEGREES

II. TWO-PART FRACTURE WHERE ONE SEGMENT IS SIGNIFICANTLY DISPLACED BY 1.0 CM OR 45 DEGREES

III. THREE-PART FRACTURE WHERE TWO SEGMENTS ARE SIGNIFICANTLY DISPLACED BY 1.0 CM OR 45 DEGREES

IV. FOUR-PART FRACTURE WHERE ALL FOUR MAJOR SEGMENTS ARE DISPLACED BY 1.0 CM OR 45 DEGREES

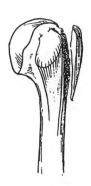

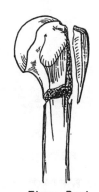

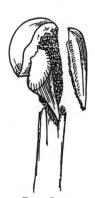

Two Part
Greater Tuberosity
Fracture

Three Part
Greater Tuberosity
and Shaft Fracture

Four Part

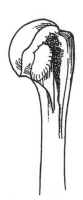

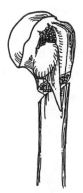

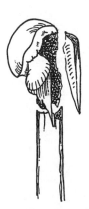

Two Part
Lesser Tuberosity
Fracture

Three Part
Lesser Tuberosity
and Shaft Fracture

Four Part

FRACTURES OF THE PROXIMAL HUMERUS

(Neer Classification)

V. FRACTURE DISLOCATION

Fracture dislocations may be ANTERIOR or POSTERIOR and are also based on the four fracture segment classification.

Classification describes only displaced segments by 1.0 cm or 45 degree angulation.

Anterior Fracture Dislocations

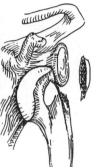

Two Part

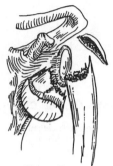

Three Part

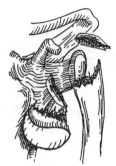

Four Part

Posterior Fracture Dislocations

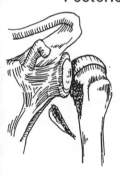

Two Part

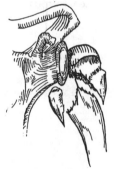

Three Part

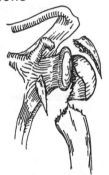

Four Part

47

FRACTURES OF THE CLAVICLE

(Anatomic Location)

I.   INNER-THIRD - 5%[a]

II. MID-THIRD - 80%

III. DISTAL-THIRD OR INTERLIGAMENTOUS - 15%

DISTAL CLAVICLE FRACTURES are further subdivided on the next page.

[a] *Percentages indicate the frequency of fracture occurrence.*

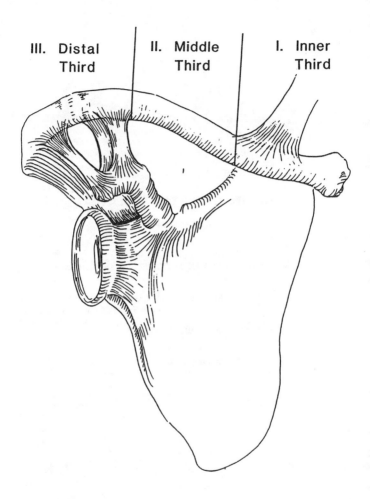

III. Distal
Third

II. Middle
Third

I. Inner
Third

49

FRACTURES OF THE DISTAL CLAVICLE

(Neer Classification)

I. INTACT LIGAMENTS WITHOUT SIGNIFICANT DISPLACEMENT

II. DISPLACED INTERLIGAMENTOUS FRACTURE WHERE CORACOCLAVICULAR LIGAMENTS ARE DETACHED FROM THE MEDIAL SEGMENT AND TRAPEZOID LIGAMENTS REMAIN ATTACHED TO THE DISTAL SEGMENT

III. ARTICULAR SURFACE FRACTURES

I.

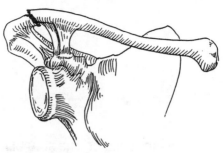

II.

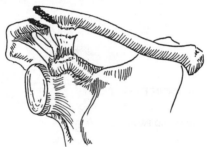

III.

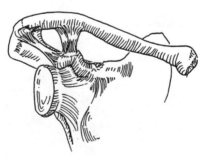

FRACTURES OF THE SCAPULA

(Anatomic Location)

I. NECK

II. ACROMIUM PROCESS

III. COROCOID PROCESS

IV. BODY

V. GLENOID RIM OR ARTICULAR SURFACE

VI. SPINOUS PROCESS

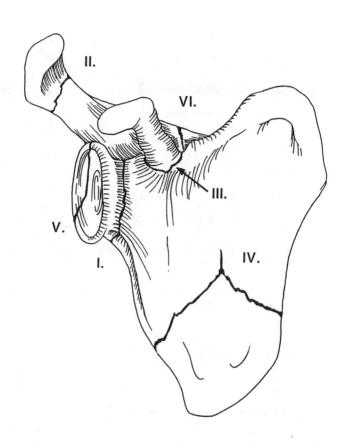

GLENOID FRACTURES

(Ideberg Classification)

I. FRACTURE OF THE ANTERIOR GLENOID MARGIN; ASSOCIATED WITH GLENOHUMERAL FRACTURE DISLOCATION

II. TRANSVERSE OR OBLIQUE FRACTURE THROUGH THE GLENOID FOSSA; MAY BE ASSOCIATED WITH INFERIOR HUMERAL HEAD SUBLUXATION OR DISLOCATION

III. OBLIQUE GLENOID FRACTURE THAT COURSES CEPHALAD TO THE MID PORTION OF THE SCAPULA

IV. HORIZONTAL FRACTURE THROUGH THE SCAPULA INVOLVING THE GLENOID FOSSA, NECK, AND BODY

V. HORIZONTAL FRACTURE COMBINED WITH TRANSVERSE COMPONENT INVOLVING THE ENTIRE SCAPULAR NECK OR JUST THE INFERIOR PORTION

Type I GLENOID FRACTURES are the most common.

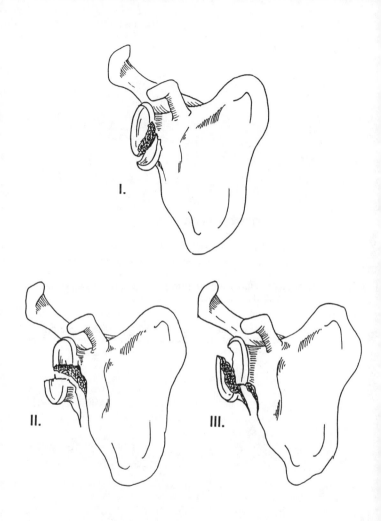

GLENOID FRACTURES

(Ideberg Classification)

IV.   HORIZONTAL FRACTURE THROUGH THE SCAPULA INVOLVING THE GLENOID FOSSA, NECK, AND BODY

V.   HORIZONTAL FRACTURE COMBINED WITH TRANSVERSE COMPONENT INVOLVING THE ENTIRE SCAPULAR NECK OR JUST THE INFERIOR PORTION

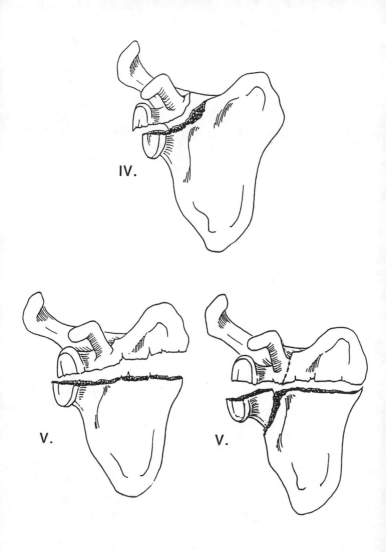

IV.

V.

V.

SPINE

CLASSIFICATION OF CERVICAL SPINE INJURIES

(Harris Classification)

I. FLEXION

    A. ANTERIOR SUBLUXATION

    B. BILATERAL INTERFACETAL DISLOCATION

    C. SIMPLE WEDGE (COMPRESSION) FRACTURE

    D. CLAY-SHOVELER (COAL-SHOVELER) FRACTURE

    E. FLEXION TEARDROP FRACTURE

II. FLEXION-ROTATION: UNILATERAL INTERFACETAL DISLOCATION

III. EXTENSION-ROTATION: PILLAR FRACTURE

IV. VERTICAL COMPRESSION

    A. JEFFERSON BURST FRACTURE OF ATLAS

    B. BURST FRACTURE

V. HYPEREXTENSION

    A. HYPEREXTENSION DISLOCATION

    B. AVULSION FRACTURE OF ANTERIOR ARCH OF THE ATLAS

    C. EXTENSION TEARDROP FRACTURE OF THE AXIS

    D. FRACTURE OF THE POSTERIOR ARCH OF THE ATLAS

    E. LAMINAR FRACTURE

    F. TRAUMATIC SPONDYLOLISTHESIS (HANGMAN'S FRACTURE)

    G. HYPEREXTENSION FRACTURE DISLOCATION

VI. LATERAL FLEXION: UNCINATE PROCESS FRACTURE

VII. DIVERSE, OR IMPRECISELY UNDERSTOOD, MECHANISMS

    A. ATLANTA-OCCIPITAL DISASSOCIATION

    B. ODONTOID FRACTURES

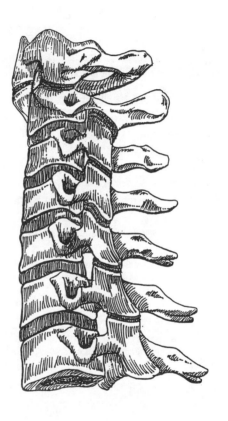

CLASSIFICATION OF CERVICAL SPINE INJURIES

(Harris Classification)

I.   FLEXION

   A.   ANTERIOR SUBLUXATION

   B.   BILATERAL INTERFACETAL DISLOCATION

   C.   SIMPLE WEDGE (COMPRESSION) FRACTURE

   D.   CLAY-SHOVELER (COAL-SHOVELER) FRACTURE

   E.   FLEXION TEARDROP FRACTURE

Additional descriptions of CLAY-SHOVELER FRACTURE in the EPONYM SECTION.

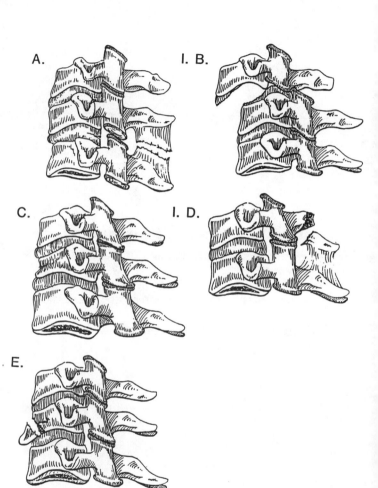

A.

I. B.

C.

I. D.

E.

63

CLASSIFICATION OF CERVICAL SPINE INJURIES

(Harris Classification)

II.   FLEXION-ROTATION: UNILATERAL INTERFACETAL DISLOCATION

III.   EXTENSION-ROTATION: PILLAR FRACTURE

II.

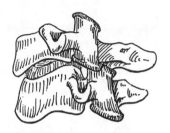

III.

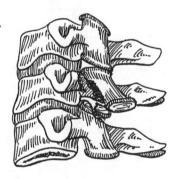

CLASSIFICATION OF CERVICAL SPINE INJURIES

(Harris Classification)

IV. VERTICAL COMPRESSION

    A.   JEFFERSON BURST FRACTURE OF ATLAS

    B.   BURST FRACTURE

IV. A.

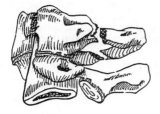 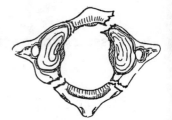

Lateral View   Axial View

IV. B.

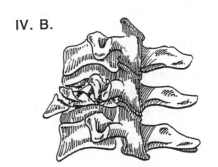

CLASSIFICATION OF CERVICAL SPINE INJURIES

(Harris Classification)

V.   HYPEREXTENSION

    A.   HYPEREXTENSION DISLOCATION

    B.   AVULSION FRACTURE OF ANTERIOR ARCH OF THE ATLAS

    C.   EXTENSION TEARDROP FRACTURE OF THE AXIS

    D.   FRACTURE OF THE POSTERIOR ARCH OF THE ATLAS

    E.   LAMINAR FRACTURE

    F.   TRAUMATIC SPONDYLOLISTHESIS (HANGMAN'S FRACTURE)

    G.   HYPERXTENSION FRACTURE DISLOCATION

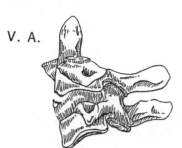

V. A.

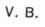

V. B.

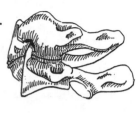

V. C.

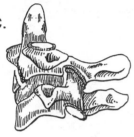

V. D.

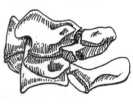

V. E.

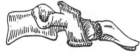

V. F.

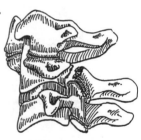

V. G.

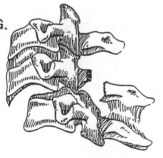

CLASSIFICATION OF CERVICAL SPINE INJURIES

(Harris Classification)

VI. LATERAL FLEXION: UNCINATE PROCESS FRACTURE

VII. DIVERSE, OR IMPRECISELY UNDERSTOOD, MECHANISMS

A. ATLANTA-OCCIPITAL DISASSOCIATION

B. ODONTOID FRACTURES

ODONTOID FRACTURE classification is located on the next page.

VI.

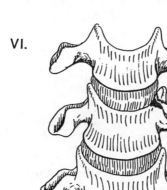

VII. A.

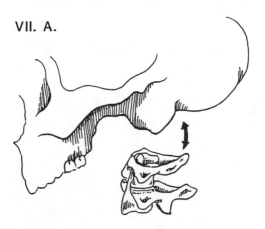

FRACTURES OF THE ODONTOID PROCESS

(Anderson and D'Alonzo Classification)

I. OBLIQUE FRACTURE THROUGH THE SUPERIOR PART OF THE ODONTOID

II. FRACTURE AT THE JUNCTION OF THE ODONTOID PROCESS AND THE AXIS

III. FRACTURE EXTENDS INTO THE BODY OF THE AXIS

ODONTOID FRACTURES may be further classified as DISPLACED or NONDISPLACED.

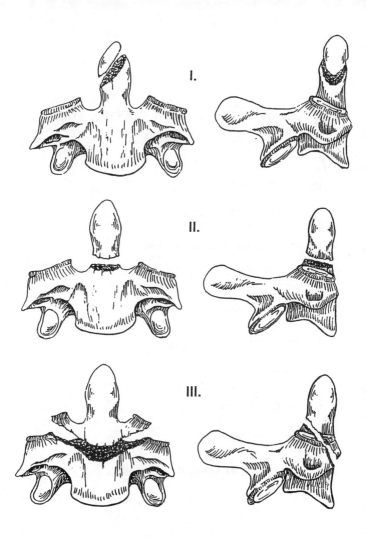

I.

II.

III.

THORACOLUMBAR SPINAL INJURY CLASSIFICATION

(Denis Classification)

I.   MINOR SPINAL INJURIES

   A.   ARTICULAR PROCESS FRACTURE

   B.   TRANSVERSE PROCESS FRACTURE

   C.   SPINOUS PROCESS FRACTURE

   D.   PARS INTERARTICULARIS FRACTURE

II. MAJOR SPINAL INJURIES

   A.   COMPRESSION FRACTURE

   B.   BURST FRACTURES

   C.   FRACTURE DISLOCATIONS

   D.   SEAT-BELT TYPE SPINAL INJURIES

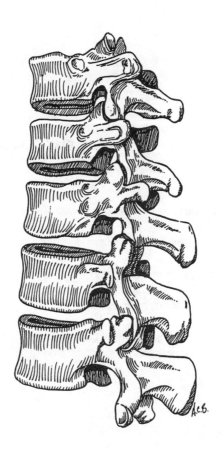

THORACOLUMBAR SPINAL INJURY CLASSIFICATION

(Denis Classification)

I.   MINOR SPINAL INJURIES

    A.   TRANSVERSE PROCESS FRACTURE

    B.   ARTICULAR PROCESS FRACTURE

    C.   SPINOUS PROCESS FRACTURE

    D.   PARS INTERARTICULARIS FRACTURE

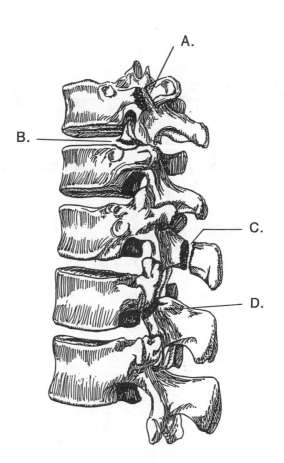

THORACOLUMBAR SPINAL INJURY CLASSIFICATION

(Denis Classification)

II.   MAJOR SPINAL INJURIES

    A.   COMPRESSION FRACTURE

    B.   BURST FRACTURES

BURST FRACTURES disrupt middle spinal segment and retropulse bone fragments toward the spinal canal.

II. A.

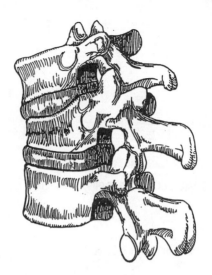

II. B.

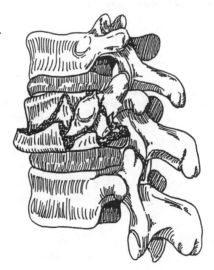

THORACOLUMBAR SPINAL INJURY CLASSIFICATION

(Denis Classification)

II.   MAJOR SPINAL INJURIES

    C.   FRACTURE DISLOCATIONS

    D.   SEAT-BELT TYPE SPINAL INJURIES

SEAT-BELT TYPE SPINAL INJURIES may be through bone, ligaments or a combination. Mechanism of injury is usually a flexion distraction type force.

II. C.

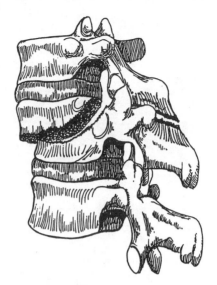

II. D.

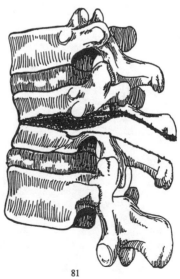

PELVIS
and
ACETABULUM

CLASSIFICATION OF PELVIC DISRUPTION

(Tile Classification)

TYPE A.   STABLE

    A1.   FRACTURES OF THE PELVIS NOT INVOLVING THE RING

    A2.   STABLE, MINIMALLY DISPLACED FRACTURES OF THE RING

TYPE B.   ROTATIONALLY UNSTABLE, VERTICALLY STABLE

    B1.   OPEN BOOK

    B2.   LATERAL COMPRESSION: IPSILATERAL

    B3.   LATERAL COMPRESSION: CONTRALATERAL (BUCKET HANDLE)

TYPE C.   ROTATIONALLY AND VERTICALLY UNSTABLE

    C1.   UNILATERAL

    C2.   BILATERAL

    C3.   ASSOCIATED WITH ACETABULAR FRACTURE

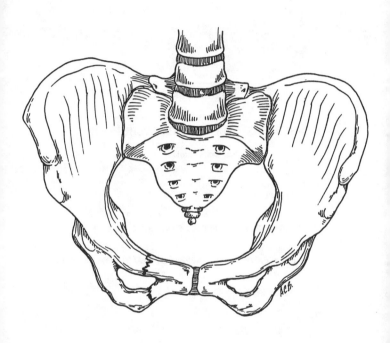

CLASSIFICATION OF PELVIC DISRUPTION

(Tile Classification)

TYPE A.   STABLE

    A1.   FRACTURES OF THE PELVIS NOT INVOLVING THE RING

    A2.   STABLE, MINIMALLY DISPLACED FRACTURES OF THE RING

A. 1.

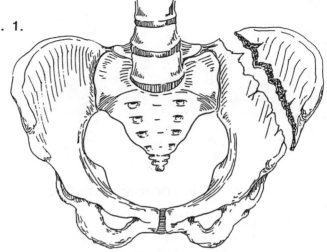

A. 2.

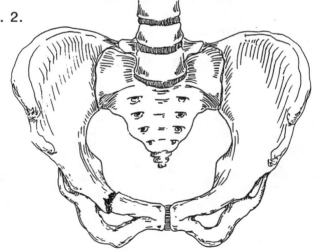

CLASSIFICATION OF PELVIC DISRUPTION

(Tile Classification)

TYPE B.   ROTATIONALLY UNSTABLE, VERTICALLY STABLE

    B1.   OPEN BOOK

    B2.   LATERAL COMPRESSION: IPSILATERAL

B. 1.

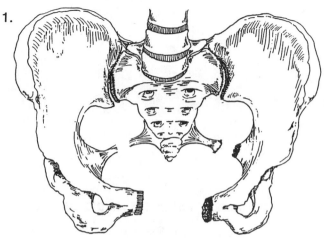

B. 2.

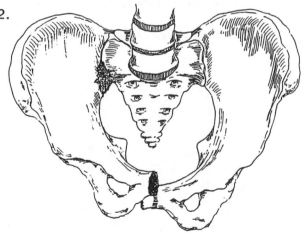

CLASSIFICATION OF PELVIC DISRUPTION

(Tile Classification)

TYPE B.   ROTATIONALLY UNSTABLE, VERTICALLY STABLE

    B3.   LATERAL COMPRESSION: CONTRALATERAL (BUCKET HANDLE)

B. 3.

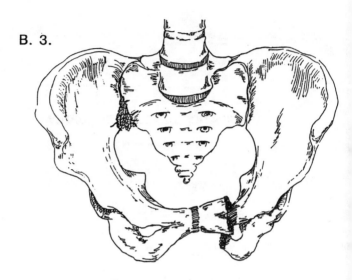

CLASSIFICATION OF PELVIC DISRUPTION

(Tile Classification)

TYPE C.   ROTATIONALLY AND VERTICALLY UNSTABLE

   C1.   UNILATERAL

   C2.   BILATERAL

   C3.   ASSOCIATED WITH ACETABULAR FRACTURE

C. 1.

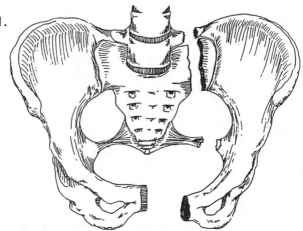

C. 2.

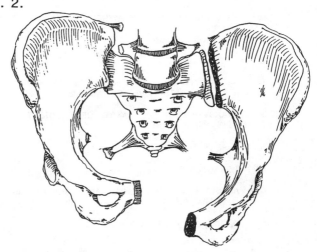

CLASSIFICATION OF ACETABULUM FRACTURES

(Tile Classification)

UNDISPLACED

DISPLACED

TYPE I. POSTERIOR TYPES WITH OR WITHOUT POSTERIOR DISLOCATION

    A. POSTERIOR COLUMN

    B. POSTERIOR WALL

        1. ASSOCIATED WITH POSTERIOR COLUMN

        2. ASSOCIATED WITH TRANSVERSE FRACTURES

TYPE II. ANTERIOR TYPES WITH OR WITHOUT ANTERIOR DISLOCATIONS

    A. ANTERIOR COLUMN

    B. ANTERIOR WALL

    C. ASSOCIATED WITH ANTERIOR WALL, ANTERIOR COLUMN, AND/OR TRANSVERSE FRACTURES

TYPE III. TRANSVERSE TYPES WITH OR WITHOUT CENTRAL DISLOCATION

    A. PURE TRANSVERSE

    B. T-FRACTURES

    C. ASSOCIATED TRANSVERSE AND ACETABULAR WALL FRACTURES

    D. DOUBLE COLUMN FRACTURES

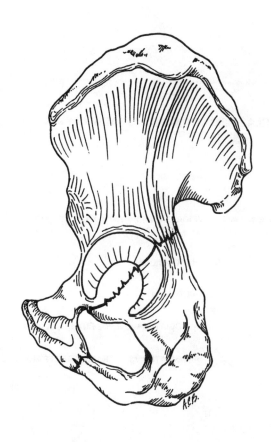

CLASSIFICATION OF ACETABULUM FRACTURES

(Tile Classification)

DISPLACED

TYPE I.   POSTERIOR TYPES WITH OR WITHOUT POSTERIOR DISLOCATION

    A.   POSTERIOR COLUMN

    B.   POSTERIOR WALL

        1.   ASSOCIATED WITH POSTERIOR COLUMN

        2.   ASSOCIATED WITH TRANSVERSE FRACTURES

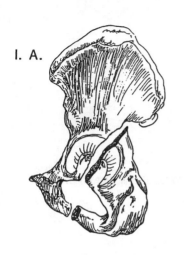

I. A.

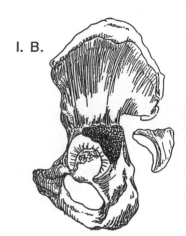

I. B.

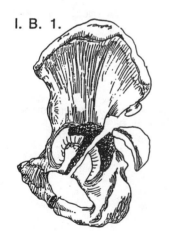

I. B. 1.

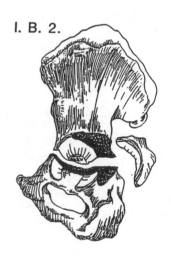

I. B. 2.

CLASSIFICATION OF ACETABULUM FRACTURES

(Tile Classification)

DISPLACED

    TYPE II.   ANTERIOR TYPES WITH OR WITHOUT ANTERIOR DISLOCATIONS

        A.   ANTERIOR COLUMN

        B.   ANTERIOR WALL

        C.   ASSOCIATED WITH ANTERIOR WALL, ANTERIOR COLUMN, AND/OR TRANSVERSE FRACTURES

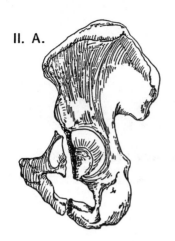

II. A.

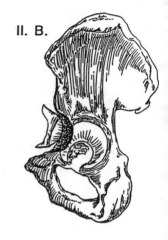

II. B.

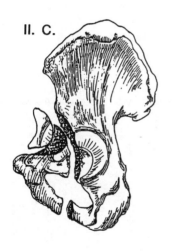

II. C.

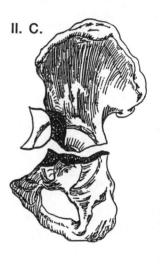

II. C.

CLASSIFICATION OF ACETABULUM FRACTURES

(Tile Classification)

DISPLACED

TYPE III.   TRANSVERSE TYPES WITH OR WITHOUT CENTRAL DISLOCATION

A.   PURE TRANSVERSE

B.   T-FRACTURES

C.   ASSOCIATED TRANSVERSE AND ACETABULAR WALL FRACTURES

D.   DOUBLE COLUMN FRACTURES

III. A.
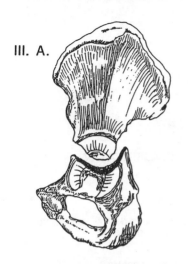

III. B.
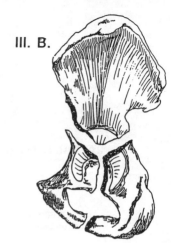

III. C.
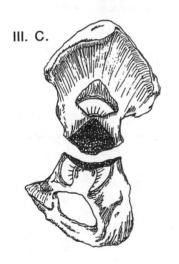

III. D.
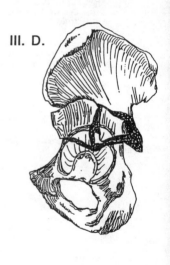

SACRAL FRACTURE CLASSIFICATION

(Denis Classification)

I. FRACTURE THROUGH SACRAL ALA WITHOUT DAMAGE TO THE CENTRAL CANAL OR SACRAL FORAMINA

II. FRACTURE INVOLVING THE SACRAL FORAMINA BUT SPARING THE CENTRAL CANAL. FRACTURE MAY ALSO INVOLVE THE ALAR ZONE

III. FRACTURE INVOLVING THE CENTRAL SACRAL CANAL. FRACTURE MAY ALSO INVOLVE FORAMINA AND ALAR ZONES

Zone II fractures are frequently associated with sciatica and nerve root injury.

Zone III fractures are frequently associated with loss of sphincter function and saddle anesthesia.

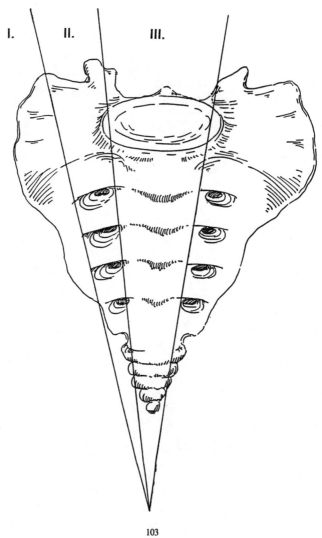

I.   II.   III.

LOWER
EXTREMITY

CLASSIFICATION OF HIP FRACTURES

(Anatomic Classification)

I. FEMORAL NECK - INTRACAPSULAR FRACTURES
    (Garden Classification)

II. INTERTROCHANTERIC - EXTRACAPSULAR FRACTURE
    (Kyle Classification)

III. SUBTROCHANTERIC
    (Seinsheimer Classification)

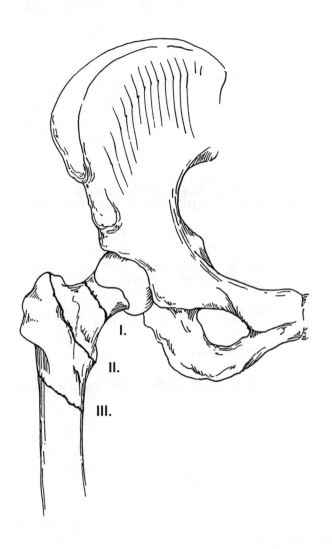

I.

II.

III.

POSTERIOR HIP DISLOCATIONS
ASSOCIATED WITH FEMORAL HEAD FRACTURES

(Pipkin Classification)

I.   POSTERIOR DISLOCATION WITH FRACTURE OF THE FEMORAL
     HEAD CAUDAD TO THE FOVEA CENTRALIS

II. POSTERIOR DISLOCATION WITH FRACTURE OF THE FEMORAL
     HEAD CEPHALAD TO THE FOVEA CENTRALIS

III. TYPE I OR II WITH FEMORAL NECK FRACTURE

IV. TYPE I, II, OR III WITH ASSOCIATED ACETABULUM FRACTURE

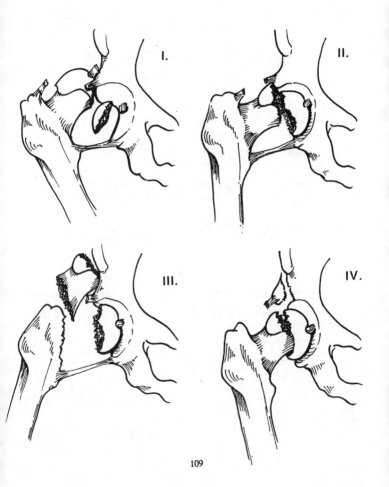

109

FRACTURES OF THE FEMORAL NECK

(Garden Classification)

I.   INCOMPLETE OR IMPACTED FRACTURE

II.   COMPLETE FRACTURE WITHOUT DISPLACEMENT

III.   COMPLETE FRACTURE WITH PARTIAL DISPLACEMENT
          (HIP CAPSULE USUALLY PARTIALLY INTACT)

IV.   COMPLETE FRACTURE WITH FULL DISPLACEMENT
          (HIP CAPSULE USUALLY COMPLETELY DISRUPTED)

Greater fracture displacement increases the incidence of avascular necrosis.

Type I femoral neck fractures may present with coxa valgus, while type III fractures demonstrate coxa varus.

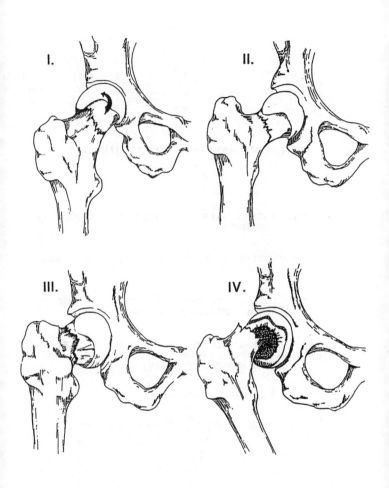

INTERTROCHANTERIC HIP FRACTURES

(Kyle Classification)

I.   NONDISPLACED STABLE INTERTROCHANTERIC FRACTURE WITHOUT COMMINUTION

II. DISPLACED STABLE INTERTROCHANTERIC FRACTURE WITH MINIMAL COMMINUTION

III. DISPLACED UNSTABLE INTERTROCHANTERIC FRACTURE WITH EXTENSIVE POSTERIOR MEDIAL COMMINUTION

IV. DISPLACED UNSTABLE INTERTROCHANTERIC FRACTURE WITH EXTENSIVE POSTERIOR MEDIAL COMMINUTION AND A SUBTROCHANTERIC COMPONENT

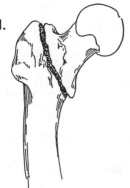

I.

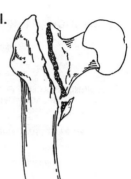

II.

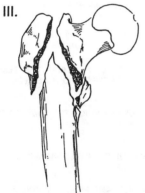

III.

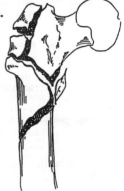

IV.

SUBTROCHANTERIC FRACTURES OF THE FEMUR

(Seinsheimer Classification)

I. NONDISPLACED FRACTURE WITH LESS THAN 2 MM OF DISPLACEMENT

II. TWO-PART FRACTURES

    IIA. TWO-PART TRANSVERSE FEMORAL FRACTURE

    IIB. TWO-PART SPIRAL FRACTURE WITH LESSER TROCHANTER ATTACHED TO PROXIMAL FRAGMENT

    IIC. TWO-PART SPIRAL FRACTURE WITH LESSER TROCHANTER ATTACHED TO DISTAL FRAGMENT

III. THREE-PART FRACTURES

    IIIA. THREE-PART SPIRAL FRACTURE IN WHICH THE LESSER TROCHANTER IS PART OF THE THIRD FRAGMENT

    IIIB. THREE-PART SPIRAL FRACTURE IN WHICH THE THIRD PART IS A BUTTERFLY FRAGMENT

IV. COMMINUTED FRACTURE WITH FOUR OR MORE FRAGMENTS

V. SUBTROCHANTERIC INTERTROCHANTERIC FRACTURE, ANY SUBTROCHANTERIC FRACTURE WITH EXTENSION THROUGH THE GREATER TROCHANTER

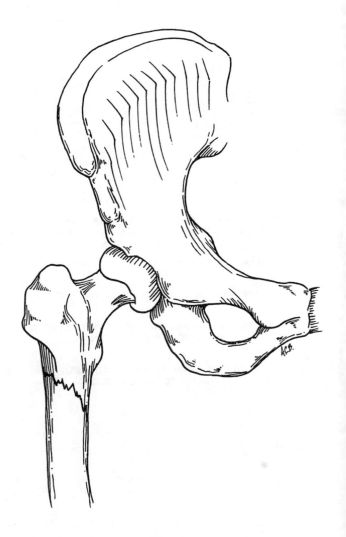

115

SUBTROCHANTERIC FRACTURES OF THE FEMUR

(Seinsheimer Classification)

I.   NONDISPLACED FRACTURE WITH LESS THAN 2 MM OF DISPLACEMENT

II.   TWO-PART FRACTURES

    IIA.   TWO-PART TRANSVERSE FEMORAL FRACTURE

    IIB.   TWO-PART SPIRAL FRACTURE WITH LESSER TROCHANTER ATTACHED TO PROXIMAL FRAGMENT

    IIC.   TWO-PART SPIRAL FRACTURE WITH LESSER TROCHANTER ATTACHED TO DISTAL FRAGMENT

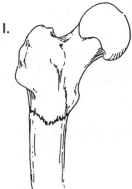

I.

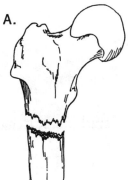

II. A.

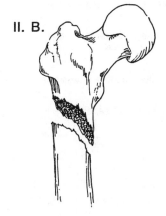

II. B.

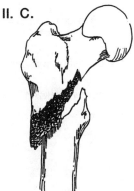

II. C.

117

SUBTROCHANTERIC FRACTURES OF THE FEMUR

(Seinsheimer Classification)

III.   THREE-PART FRACTURES

    IIIA.   THREE-PART SPIRAL FRACTURE IN WHICH THE LESSER TROCHANTER IS PART OF THE THIRD FRAGMENT

    IIIB.   THREE-PART SPIRAL FRACTURE IN WHICH THE THIRD PART IS A BUTTERFLY FRAGMENT

IV.   COMMINUTED FRACTURE WITH FOUR OR MORE FRAGMENTS

V.   SUBTROCHANTERIC - INTERTROCHANTERIC FRACTURE

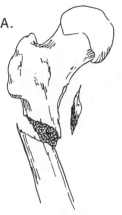

III. A.

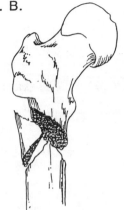

III. B.

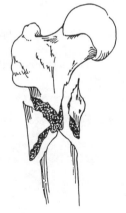

IV.

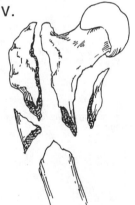

V.

FEMORAL SHAFT FRACTURES

(Winquist Classification of Comminution)

I.   FEMORAL SHAFT FRACTURE WITH VERY SMALL BUTTERFLY FRAGMENT (25% OR LESS OF THE WIDTH OF THE BONE)

II.   COMMINUTED FEMORAL SHAFT FRACTURE WITH BUTTERFLY FRAGMENT 50% OR LESS OF THE WIDTH OF THE BONE

III.   COMMINUTED FRACTURE WITH LARGE BUTTERFLY SEGMENT GREATER THAN 50% OF THE WIDTH OF THE BONE

IV.   SEVERE COMMINUTION OF AN ENTIRE SEGMENT OF BONE

V.   FEMORAL SHAFT FRACTURE WITH SEGMENTAL BONE LOSS

Increasing comminution decreases inherent stability to rotation, shortening, and angulation.

120

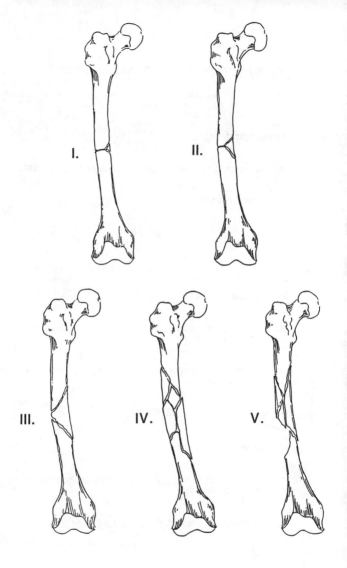

I. II.

III. IV. V.

121

SUPRACONDYLAR FEMORAL FRACTURES

(AO Classification)

A. EXTRA-ARTICULAR

   A1. AVULSION OF THE MEDIAL OR LATERAL EPICONDYLE

   A2. SIMPLE SUPRACONDYLAR

   A3. COMMINUTED SUPRACONDYLAR

B. UNICONDYLAR

   B1. MEDIAL OR LATERAL CONDYLE

   B2. CONDYLE FRACTURE WITH EXTENSION PROXIMALLY INTO FEMORAL SHAFT

   B3. POSTERIOR TANGENTIAL FRACTURE OF ONE OR BOTH CONDYLES

C. BICONDYLAR

   C1. INTERCONDYLAR

   C2. INTERCONDYLAR WITH A COMMINUTED SUPRACONDYLAR COMPONENT

   C3. SEVERLY COMMINUTED BICONDYLAR FRACTURE

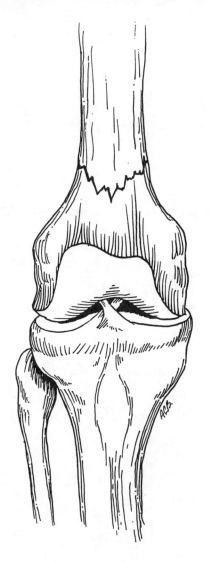

SUPRACONDYLAR FEMORAL FRACTURES

(AO Classification)

A. EXTRA-ARTICULAR

    A1. AVULSION OF THE MEDIAL OR LATERAL EPICONDYLE

    A2. SIMPLE SUPRACONDYLAR

    A3. COMMINUTED SUPRACONDYLAR

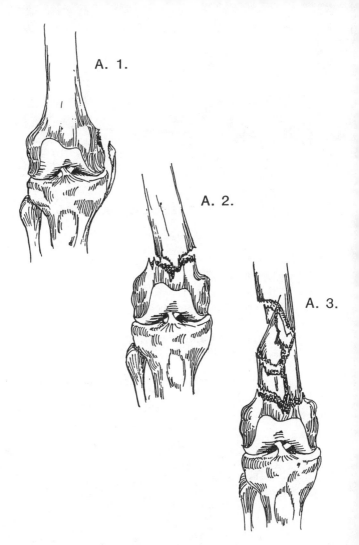

A. 1.

A. 2.

A. 3.

125

SUPRACONDYLAR FEMORAL FRACTURES

(AO Classification)

B. UNICONDYLAR

B1. MEDIAL OR LATERAL CONDYLE

B2. CONDYLE FRACTURE WITH EXTENSION PROXIMALLY INTO FEMORAL SHAFT

B3. POSTERIOR TANGENTIAL FRACTURE OF ONE OR BOTH CONDYLES

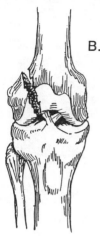

B. 1.

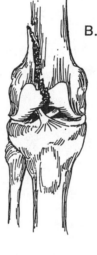

B. 2.

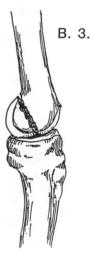

B. 3.

127

SUPRACONDYLAR FEMORAL FRACTURES

(AO Classification)

C. BICONDYLAR

    C1. INTERCONDYLAR

    C2. INTERCONDYLAR WITH A COMMINUTED SUPRACONDYLAR COMPONENT

    C3. SEVERLY COMMINUTED BICONDYLAR FRACTURE

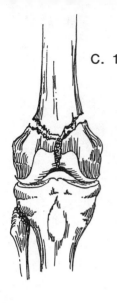

C. 1.

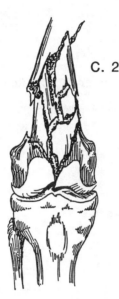

C. 2.

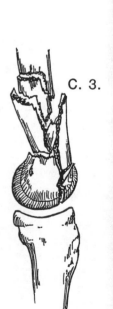

C. 3.

PATELLA FRACTURES

(Fracture Configuration Classification)

I.   NONDISPLACED

II. TRANSVERSE

III. UPPER OR LOWER POLE

IV. COMMINUTED

V.   VERTICAL

I.

II.

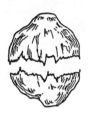

III.

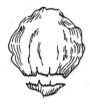

IV.

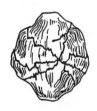

V.

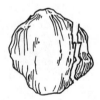

FRACTURES OF THE TIBIAL SPINE

(Meyers Classification)

I. FRACTURE TILTED UP ONLY ANTERIORLY

II. ANTERIOR PORTION LIFTED COMPLETELY FROM TIBIA WITH ONLY SOME POSTERIOR ATTACHMENT

IIIA. INTERCONDYLAR FRAGMENT NOT IN CONTACT WITH THE TIBIA

IIIB. INTERCONDYLAR FRAGMENT ROTATED

I.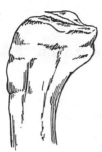

II.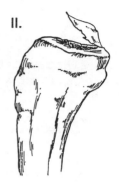

III. A.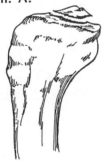

III. B.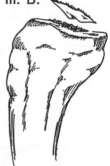

FRACTURES OF THE TIBIAL PLATEAU

(Schatzker Classification)

I.   CLEAVAGE OR WEDGE TYPE FRACTURES OF THE LATERAL TIBIAL PLATEAU - 24%[a]

II.   LATERAL WEDGE FRACTURE WITH ADJACENT DEPRESSION - 26%

III. PURE CENTRAL DEPRESSION WITHOUT AN ASSOCIATED WEDGE FRACTURE - 26%

IV.   WEDGE OR DEPRESSION FRACTURES OF THE MEDIAL TIBIAL PLATEAU - 11%

V.   BICONDYLAR FRACTURE OF THE TIBIAL PLATEAU - 10%

VI.   TIBIAL PLATEAU FRACTURE WITH DISASSOCIATION OF THE METAPHYSIS FROM THE DIAPHYSIS BY A FRACTURE - 3%

[a] *Percentages indicate the frequency of fracture occurrence.*

134

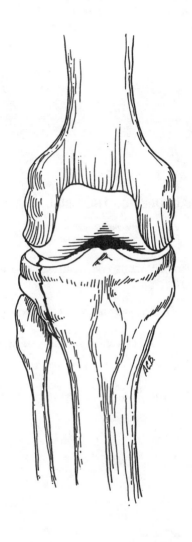

FRACTURES OF THE TIBIAL PLATEAU

(Schatzker Classification)

I. CLEAVAGE OR WEDGE TYPE FRACTURES OF THE LATERAL TIBIAL PLATEAU

II. LATERAL WEDGE FRACTURE WITH ADJACENT DEPRESSION

III. PURE CENTRAL DEPRESSION WITHOUT AN ASSOCIATED WEDGE FRACTURE

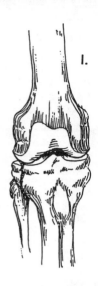

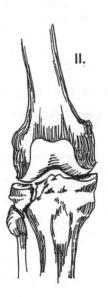

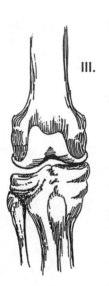

FRACTURES OF THE TIBIAL PLATEAU

(Schatzker Classification)

IV.   WEDGE OR DEPRESSION FRACTURES OF THE MEDIAL TIBIAL PLATEAU

V.   BICONDYLAR FRACTURE OF THE TIBIAL PLATEAU

VI.   TIBIAL PLATEAU FRACTURE WITH DISASSOCIATION OF THE METAPHYSIS FROM THE DIAPHYSIS BY A FRACTURE

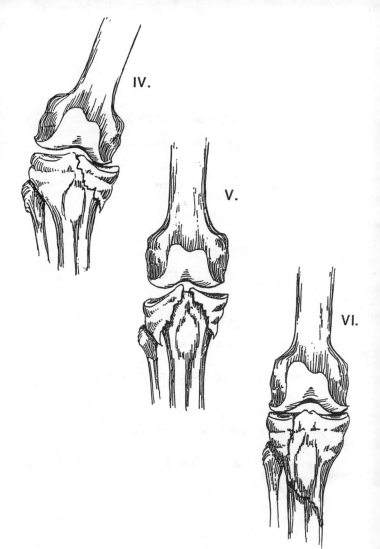

IV.

V.

VI.

TIBIAL SHAFT FRACTURES

(Chapman Classification)

A. TRANSVERSE OR SHORT OBLIQUE

B. SMALL BUTTERFLY FRAGMENT

C. LARGE BUTTERFLY FRAGMENT

D. SEGMENTAL COMMINUTION

E. SPIRAL

F. PROMIMAL ONE-FOURTH TRANSVERSE OR OBLIQUE

G. DISTAL ONE-FOURTH TRANSVERSE OR OBLIQUE

Type A is usually stable; B and C stability depend on the size of the butterfly fragment.

Type D is usually unstable while types E, F and G are stable but difficult to control.

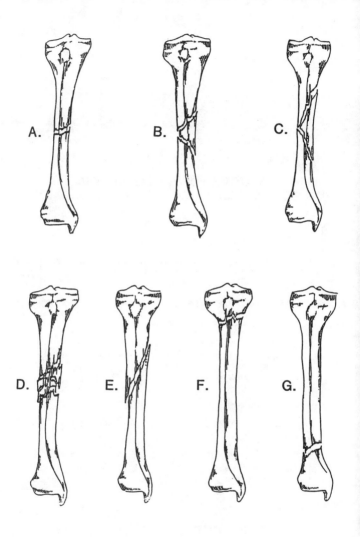

FRACTURES OF THE DISTAL TIBIA
WITH INTRA-ARTICULAR EXTENSION - PILON FRACTURE

(AO Classification)

I. CLEAVAGE FRACTURES OF THE ARTICULAR SURFACE WITHOUT
    SIGNIFICANT DISPLACEMENT

II. CLEAVAGE FRACTURES OF THE ARTICULAR SURFACE WITH
    SIGNIFICANT ARTICULAR INCONGRUITY, BUT WITHOUT
    EXTENSIVE COMMINUTION

III. CLEAVAGE FRACTURES OF THE ARTICULAR SURFACE WITH
     SIGNIFICANT COMPRESSION, DISPLACEMENT, AND
     COMMINUTION

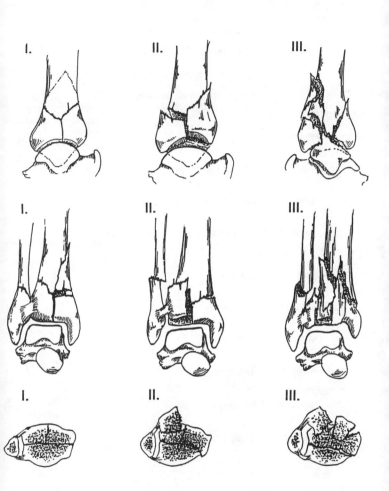

I. II. III.

I. II. III.

I. II. III.

ANKLE FRACTURE CLASSIFICATIONS[a]

(AO Classification)

(Lauge - Hansen Classification)

AO CLASSIFICATION

    A.   TRANSVERSE FIBULA FRACTURE AT OR BELOW JOINT LINE

    B.   SPRAL FIBULA FRACTURE BEGINNING AT JOINT LINE

    C.   OBLIQUE FIBULA FRACTURE ABOVE ANKLE MORTISE

LAUGE - HANSEN CLASSIFICATION

    A.   SUPINATION - EVERSION

    B.   SUPINATION - ADDUCTION

    C.   PRONATION - ABDUCTION

    D.   PRONATION - EVERSION

    E.   PRONATION - DORSIFLEXION

[a] *Two widely used classifications exist for ankle fractures.*

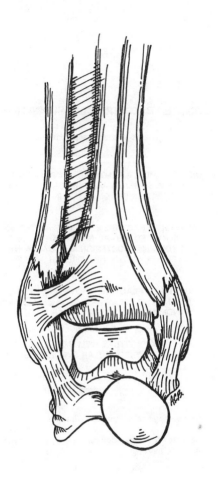

145

ANKLE FRACTURE CLASSIFICATIONS

(Danis-Weber Classification)

A. TRANSVERSE FIBULA FRACTURE AT OR BELOW THE JOINT LINE WITH POSSIBLE SHEAR FRACTURE OF THE MEDIAL MALLEOLUS. TIBIOFIBULAR SYNDESMOSIS INTACT.

B. SPIRAL FIBULA FRACTURE BEGINNING AT THE JOINT LINE WITH ASSOCIATED MEDIAL INJURY. ANTERIOR SYNDESMOSIS MAY BE TORN BUT POSTERIOR IS USUALLY INTACT. OVERALL INTEGRITY OF THE TIBIOFIBULAR SYNDESMOSIS IS INTACT.

C1. OBLIQUE FIBULA FRACTURE ABOVE A RUPTURED TIBIOFIBULAR LIGAMENT WITH ASSOCIATED MEDIAL INJURY. TIBIOFIBULAR SYNDESMOSIS IS ALWAYS DISRUPTED.

C2. OBIQUE FIBULA FRACTURE WELL ABOVE ANKLE MORTISE WITH EXTENSIVE TIBIOFIBULAR SYNDESMOSIS DISRUPTION.

This classification emphasizes the fibula fracture.

The more proximal the fibular fracture, the greater the syndesmosis injury and displacement of the ankle mortise.

146

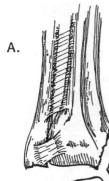

A.

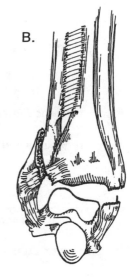

B.

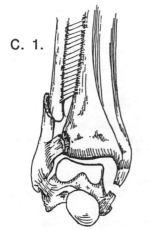

C. 1.

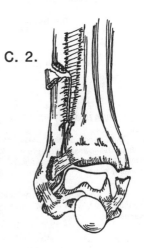

C. 2.

ANKLE FRACTURE CLASSIFICATIONS

(Lauge - Hansen Classification)

A. SUPINATION - EVERSION

    I. DISRUPTION OF THE ANTERIOR TIBIOFIBULAR LIGAMENT

    II. SPIRAL OBLIQUE FRACTURE OF THE DISTAL FIBULA

    III. DISRUPTION POSTERIOR TIBIOFIBULAR LIGAMENT, MAY FRACTURE POSTERIOR TIBIA

    IV. MEDIAL MALLEOLUS FRACTURE OR DELTOID LIGAMENT TEAR

B. SUPINATION - ADDUCTION

    I. TRANSVERSE FRACTURE LATERAL MALLEOLUS OR RUPTURE COLLATERAL LIGAMENT

    II. VERTICAL FRACTURE OF MEDIAL MALLEOLUS

SUPINATION - EVERSION is the most common type.

The Lauge - Hansen Classification is based on mechanism of injury. The first word in the classification refers to the position of the foot (SUPINATION or PRONATION) at the time of injury. The second word refers to the direction of the deforming force.

Each of the four injury categories are subdivided into stages indicating increasing severity of injury. Higher stages indicate more severe injury and worse prognosis.

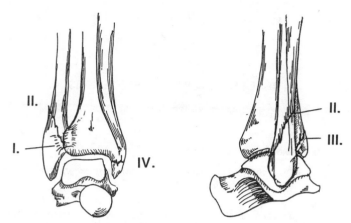

A. Supination Eversion

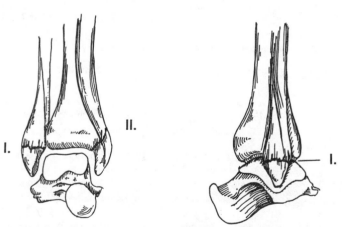

B. Supination Adduction

ANKLE FRACTURE CLASSIFICATIONS

(Lauge - Hansen Classification)

C. PRONATION - ABDUCTION

    I. TRANSVERSE FRACTURE OF THE MEDIAL MALLEOLUS OR DELTOID LIGAMENT RUPTURE

    II. ANTERIOR AND POSTURE TIBIOFIBULAR LIGAMENT RUPTURE WITH OR WITHOUT FRAGMENT OF POSTERIOR MARGIN OF THE TIBIA

    III. SHORT HORIZONTALLY DIRECTED OBLIQUE FIBULA FRACTURE

D. PRONATION - EVERSION

    I. FRACTURE OF THE MEDIAL MALLEOLUS OR RUPTURE OF THE DELTOID LIGAMENT

    II. TEAR OF THE ANTERIOR TIBIOFIBULAR AND INTEROSSEOUS LIGAMENTS

    III. SPIRAL FRACTURE OF THE FIBULA 7 TO 8 CM PROXIMAL TO THE TIP OF THE LATERAL MALLEOLUS

    IV. FRACTURE OF THE POSTERIOR LIP OF THE TIBIA

150

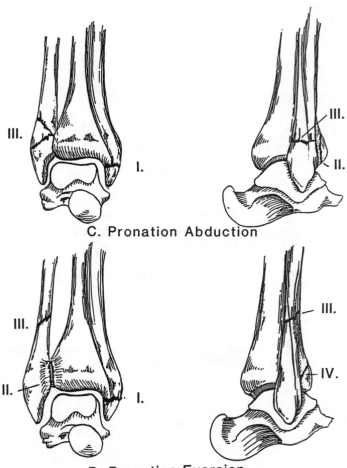

C. Pronation Abduction

D. Pronation Eversion

ANKLE FRACTURE CLASSIFICATIONS

(Lauge - Hansen Classification)

E. PRONATION - DORSIFLEXION

   I.   FRACTURE OF THE MEDIAL MALLEOLUS OR RUPTURE OF THE DELTOID LIGAMENT

   II.   ANTERIOR ARTICULAR TIBIA FRACTURE CAUSED BY DORSIFLEXION OF THE TALUS

   III. SUPRAMALLEOLAR FIBULA FRACTURE

   IV.   AVULSION FRACTURE OF THE POSTERIOR TIBIA CAUSED BY CONTINUED DORSIFLEXION OF THE TALUS

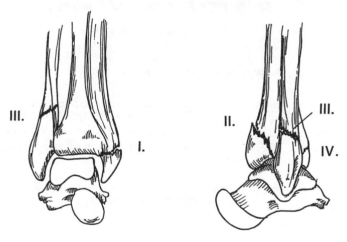

E. Pronation Dorsiflexion

FRACTURES OF THE NECK OF THE TALUS

(Modified Hawkins Classification)

I.   NONDISPLACED VERTICAL FRACTURE

II.   DISPLACED FRACTURE WITH SUBLUXATION OR DISLOCATION OF THE SUBTALAR JOINT, BUT THE ANKLE MORTISE REMAINS INTACT

III. DISPLACED FRACTURE WITH BOTH SUBTALAR AND TIBIOTALAR DISLOCATIONS

IV.   DISPLACED FRACTURE WITH DISLOCATION OF THE NECK FRAGMENT, WHILE THE BODY REMAINS REDUCED

Rate of avascular necrosis of the talus is related to the degree of fracture displacement.

Type IV fractures are rare.

No muscles or tendons originate or insert on talus.

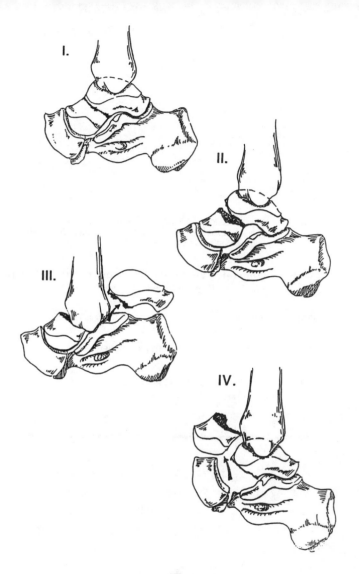

I.

II.

III.

IV.

TALAR BODY FRACTURES

(DeLee Classification)

GROUP I.   COMPRESSION OR TRANSCHONDRAL FRACTURES OF THE TALAR DOME; INCLUDES OSTEOCHONDRITIS DISSECANS OF THE TALUS

GROUP II.   CORONAL, SAGGITAL, OR HORIZONTAL SHEARING FRACTURES OF THE ENTIRE TALAR BODY

GROUP III.   POSTERIOR TUBERCLE FRACTURE OF THE TALUS

GROUP IV.   LATERAL PROCESS TALAR FRACTURE

GROUP V.   TALAR BODY CRUSH FRACTURES

Talar body fractures are uncommon and constitute approximately 1% of all fractures.

156

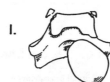

I.

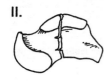 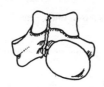 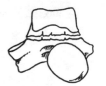

II.

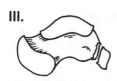

III.

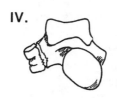

IV.

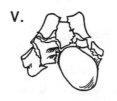

V.

FRACTURES OF THE CALCANEUS

(Essex - Lopresti Classification)

I. EXTRA-ARTICULAR FRACTURES - 25%[a]

    A. ANTERIOR PROCESS - AVULSION OR COMPRESSION

    B. TUBEROSITY

    C. MEDIAL PROCESS

    D. SUSTENACULUM TALI

    E. BODY WITHOUT INVOLVEMENT OF THE SUBTALAR JOINT

II. INTRA-ARTICULAR FRACTURES - 75%

    A. NONDISPLACED

    B. JOINT DEPRESSION

    C. TONGUE TYPE

    D. SEVERELY COMMINUTED

[a] *Percentages indicate the frequency of fracture occurrence.*

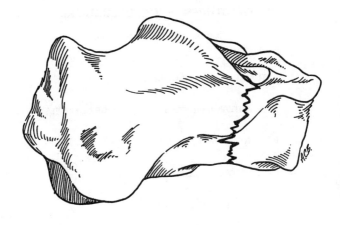

FRACTURES OF THE CALCANEUS

(Essex - Lopresti Classification)

I.   EXTRA-ARTICULAR FRACTURES - 25%

    A.   ANTERIOR PROCESS - AVULSION OR COMPRESSION

    B.   TUBEROSITY

    C.   MEDIAL PROCESS

    D.   SUSTENACULUM TALI

    E.   BODY WITHOUT INVOLVEMENT OF THE SUBTALAR JOINT

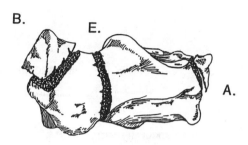

Lateral View

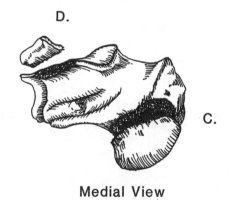

Medial View

FRACTURES OF THE CALCANEUS

(Essex - Lopresti Classification)

II.   INTRA-ARTICULAR FRACTURES - 75%

    A.   NONDISPLACED

    B.   JOINT DEPRESSION

    C.   TONGUE TYPE

    D.   SEVERELY COMMINUTED

INTRA-ARTICULAR CALCANEUS FRACTURES are frequently associated with other injuries, including ipsilateral lower extremity injuries and thoracolumbar spine fractures.

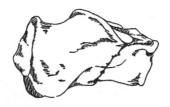

A.

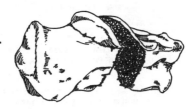

B.

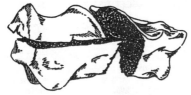

C.

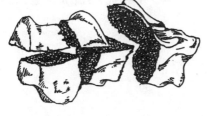

D.

163

CLASSIFICATION OF OPEN FRACTURES

(Gustilo Classification)

I.   LOW ENERGY WOUND THAT IS USUALLY LESS THAN 1 CM, OFTEN
       CAUSED BY BONE PIERCING THE SKIN

II.   WOUND GREATER THAN 1 CM IN LENGTH WITH MODERATE AMOUNT
       OF SOFT TISSUE DAMAGE SECONDARY TO HIGHER ENERGY

III.   HIGH ENERGY WOUND THAT IS USUALLY GREATER THAN 1 CM WITH
       EXTENSIVE SOFT TISSUE DAMAGE

Certain factors always constitute a Type III open fracture: high velocity gunshot wound, shotgun wound, segmental fracture, concommitant major vascular injury, significant diaphyseal bone loss, fracture occurring in a farmyard environment or by the crushing of a fast moving vehicle.

Type III fractures are further subdivided into IIIA (limited periosteal muscle stripping with adequate soft tissue coverage), IIIB (extensive soft tissue and periosteal stripping without adequate local coverage), and IIIC (associated with arterial injury requiring repair).

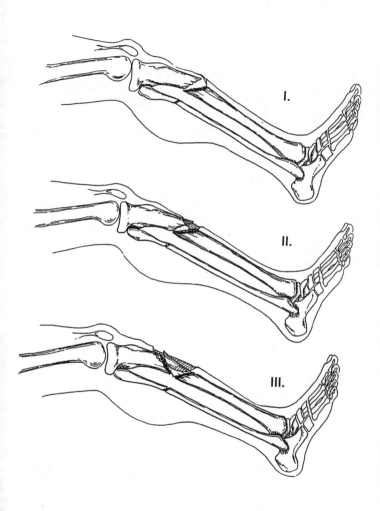

PEDIATRICS

PHYSEAL INJURIES

(Modified Salter-Harris Classification)

I.   COMPLETE SEPARATION OF THE EPIPHYSIS FROM THE METAPHYSIS WITHOUT EVIDENCE OF METAPHYSEAL FRAGMENT

II.   FRACTURE PROPAGATES ACROSS THE GROWTH PLATE FOR A DISTANCE AND EXITS THROUGH THE METAPHYSIS

III.   FRACTURE PROPAGATES ACROSS THE GROWTH PLATE AND EXITS THROUGH THE EPIPHYSIS CAUSING AN INTRA-ARTICULAR FRACTURE

IV.   VERTICAL FRACTURE THAT IS INTRA-ARTICULAR AND TRAVERSES THROUGH THE EPIPHYSIS, ACROSS THE GROWTH PLATE, AND METAPHYSIS

V.   CRUSH INJURY TO THE GROWTH PLATE

VI.   PERIPHERAL INJURY TO THE EDGE OF THE PHYSIS OR PERICHONDRAL RING

Type II is the most common fracture configuration. Metaphyseal fragmant is referred to as Thurston Holland fragment.

All growth plate fracrures require anatomic reduction to decrease chances of growth arrest.

Type V is rare.

I.

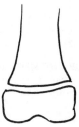

II.

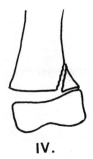

III.

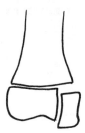

IV.

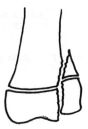

V.

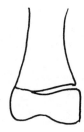

VI.

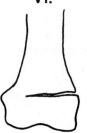

SUPRACONDYLAR FRACTURES OF THE HUMERUS

(Pirone Classification)

I.   UNDISPLACED

II.   PARTIAL DISPLACEMENT WITH CONTACT BETWEEN PROXIMAL
      AND DISTAL FRAGMENTS

      A.   POSTERIOR TILT

      B.   POSTERIOR TRANSLATION

III. COMPLETE DISPLACEMENT WITHOUT CONTACT BETWEEN THE
      PROXIMAL AND DISTAL FRAGMENTS

The same classification scheme is applicable to flexion type supracondylar fractures.

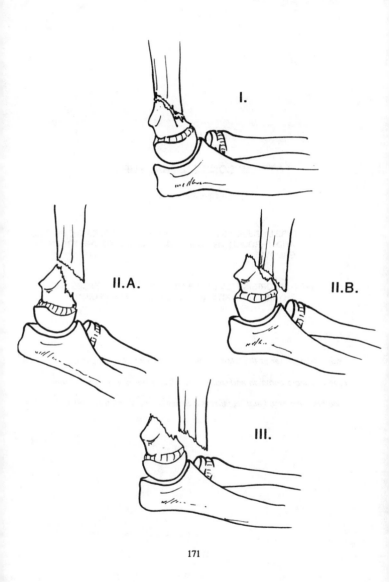

171

LATERAL CONDYLE FRACTURE

(Milch Classification)

I. FRACTURE LINE BEGINS IN THE METAPHYSIS, CROSSES THE PHYSIS, AND THROUGH THE EPIPHYSIS LATERAL TO THE TROCHLEA GROOVE

II. FRACTURE ORIGINATES IN THE METAPHYSIS, TRAVERSES THE PHYSIS, AND EXITS INTO THE TROCHLEAR REGION

Ossification center of the lateral condyle extends into the trochlea.

Type II is more common and represents a Salter-Harris II fracture pattern.

Type I is uncommon and represents a Salter-Harris IV fracture pattern.

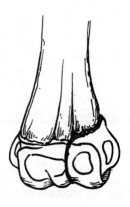

I.

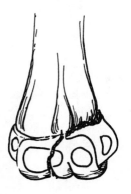

II.

MEDIAL CONDYLE FRACTURE

(Milch Classification)

I.   FRACTURE LINE ORIGINATES IN THE METAPHYSIS AND TRAVERSES
        THROUGH THE TROCHLEA NOTCH

II.   FRACTURE TRAVERSES FROM THE METAPHYSIS INTO THE
        CAPITOTROCHLEAR GROOVE

Type I is more common.

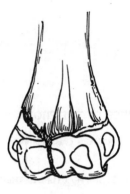

I.

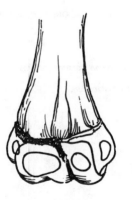

II.

FRACTURES OF THE PROXIMAL RADIUS

(Wilkins Classification)

I. SALTER-HARRIS I OR II FRACTURE OF THE PROXIMAL RADIUS PHYSIS

II. SALTER-HARRIS IV FRACTURE OF THE PROXIMAL RADIUS PHYSIS

III. METAPHYSEAL FRACTURE ONLY, WITHOUT PHYSEAL INJURY

I and II are the most common fracture patterns.

May occur with elbow dislocation.

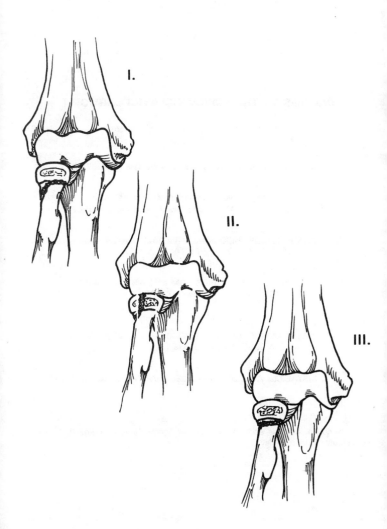

I.

II.

III.

177

INJURIES TO THE ACRIOMIOCLAVICULAR JOINT

(Dameron and Rockwood Classification)

I. MILD SPRAIN WITHOUT DISRUPTION OF THE PERIOSTEUM

II. PARTIAL DISRUPTION OF THE DORSAL PERIOSTEUM
     WITH SOME ABNORMAL DISTAL CLAVICLE MOBILITY

III. DISRUPTION OF THE DORSAL PERIOSTEUM WITH GROSS
      INSTABILITY OF THE DISTAL CLAVICLE

IV. DISRUPTION OF THE PERIOSTEUM AND DISTAL CLAVICLE
     POSTERIOR INTO, AND OCCASIONALLY, THROUGH THE
     TRAPEZIUS MUSCLE

V. SEVERE DISRUPTION OF THE PERIOSTEUM AND DISTAL CLAVICLE
    TO A SUBCUTANEOUS POSITION

VI. DISTAL CLAVICLE DISPLACED BENEATH THE COROCOID PROCESS

Acriomioclavicular and coracoclavicular ligaments remain attached to the periosteum of the clavicle.

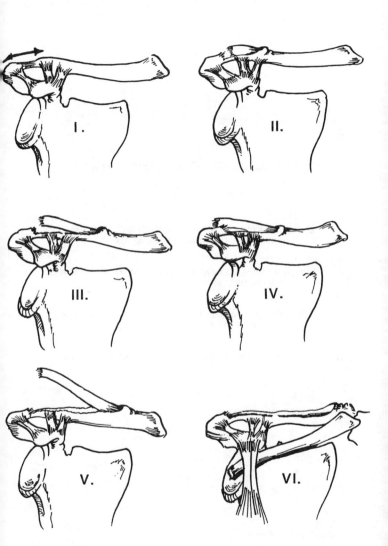

ATLANTOAXIAL ROTATORY DISPLACEMENT

(Fielding Classification)

I.   SIMPLE ROTATORY DISPLACEMENT WITH ANTERIOR SHIFT OF THE FIRST CERVICAL VERTEBRAE (C1)

II.   ROTATORY DISPLACEMENT OF C1 WITH AN ANTERIOR SHIFT OF 5 MM OR LESS

III.   ROTATORY DISPLACEMENT OF C1 WITH AN ANTERIOR SHIFT OF GREATER THAN 5 MM

IV.   ROTATORY DISPLACEMENT OF C1 WITH A POSTERIOR SHIFT

Type I is the most common.

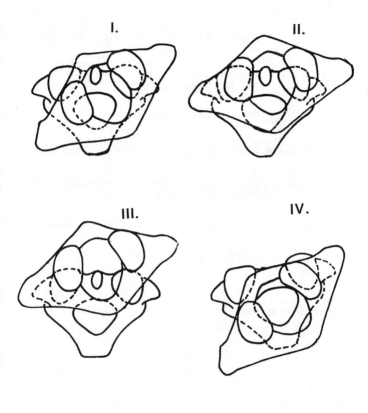

I.

II.

III.

IV.

181

HIP FRACTURES

(Delbet and Colonna Classification)

I. TRANSEPIPHYSEAL FRACTURES — THROUGH THE GROWTH PLATE

II. TRANSCERVICAL FRACTURES — BETWEEN THE EPIPHYSEAL PLATE
    AND THE BASE OF THE NECK

III. CERVICOTROCHANTERIC FRACTURE — BASE OF THE FEMORAL NECK

IV. INTERTROCHANTERIC OR PERITROCHANTERIC

Type II is the most common.

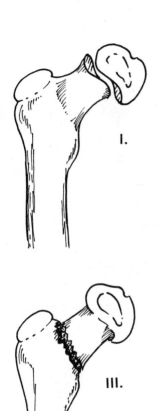

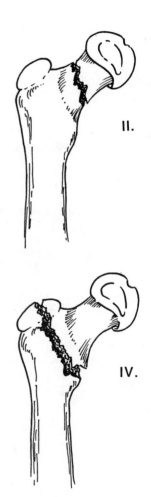

AVULSIONS OF THE TIBIAL TUBERCLE

(Watson Jones Classification)

I.   TIBIAL TUBERCLE AVULSED AND HINGED UPWARD WITHOUT
      DISPLACEMENT OF THE BASE

II.   TIBIAL TUBERCLE AVULSED AND HINGE FRACTURES WITH
      RETRACTION IN A PROXIMAL DIRECTION

III. TIBIAL TUBERCLE AND PORTION OF THE ARTICULAR SURFACE
      INCLUDED

Type III is a Salter-Harris IV fracture.

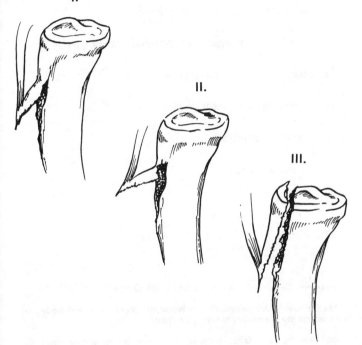

I.

II.

III.

DISTAL TIBIA AND FIBULA PHYSEAL FRACTURES

(Dias and Tachdjian Classification)

I.   SUPINATION — EXTERNAL ROTATION (SER)

II.   PRONATION — EVERSION AND EXTERNAL ROTATION (PEER)

III.   SUPINATION — PLANTAR FLEXION (SPF)

IV.   SUPINATION — INVERSION (SI)

V.   AXIAL COMPRESSION

VI.   JUVENILE TILLAUX

VII.   TRIPLANE

VIII. OTHER

Combines the Lauge-Hansen principles and the Salter-Harris classification.

The first word in the classification represents the foot position and the second phrase indicates the direction of the disrupting force.

Reduction maneuver is accomplished by reversing the disrupting force.

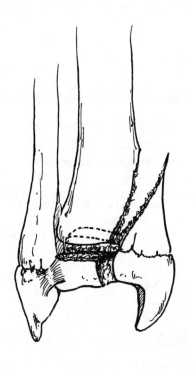

DISTAL TIBIA AND FIBULA PHYSEAL FRACTURES

(Dias and Tachdjian Classification)

I.   SUPINATION — EXTERNAL ROTATION (SER)

        STAGE I. SALTER-HARRIS I OR II WITH LONG SPIRAL DISTAL
                    TIBIAL METAPHYSEAL LOCATED POSTERIORLY

        STAGE II. SPIRAL FRACTURE OF THE FIBULA OR SALTER-HARRIS
                    FRACTURE

I.

Stage

I.

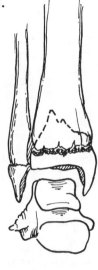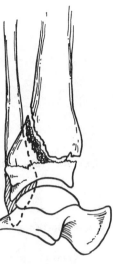

Stage

II.

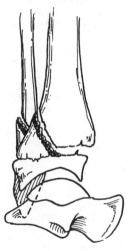

DISTAL TIBIA AND FIBULA PHYSEAL FRACTURES

(Dias and Tachdjian Classification)

II.   PRONATION — EVERSION AND EXTERNAL ROTATION (PEER)

      SALTER-HARRIS II FRACTURE OF THE TIBIA WITH SHORT
           FIBULAR FRACTURE 4 TO 7 CM FROM THE LATERAL
           MALLEOLUS

III.   SUPINATION — PLANTAR FLEXION (SPF)

      SALTER-HARRIS II FRACTURE OF THE DISTAL TIBIA VISUALIZED
           ON LATERAL X-RAY

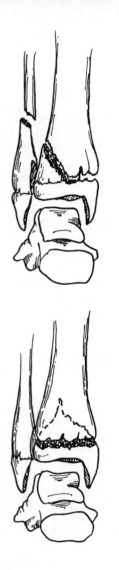

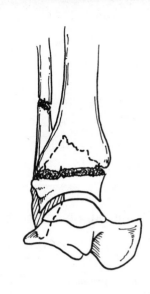

II.

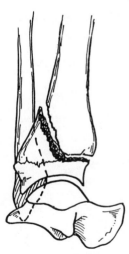

III.

DISTAL TIBIA AND FIBULA PHYSEAL FRACTURES

(Dias and Tachdjian Classification)

IV.   SUPINATION — INVERSION (SI)

STAGE I.   SALTER-HARRIS I OR II FRACTURE OF THE
            DISTAL FIBULA PHYSIS FROM TRACTION

STAGE II.   SALTER-HARRIS III OR IV THE DISTAL MEDIAL
             TIBIA

IV.

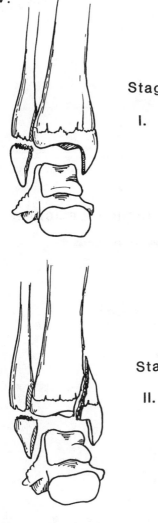

Stage

I.

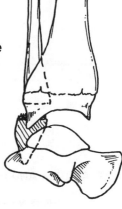

Stage

II.

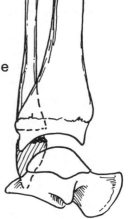

DISTAL TIBIA AND FIBULA PHYSEAL FRACTURES

(Dias and Tachdjian Classification)

V.   AXIAL COMPRESSION

DIRECT LOAD TO THE TIBIAL PHYSIS

V.

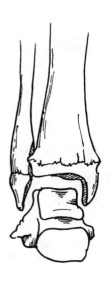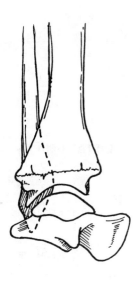

DISTAL TIBIA AND FIBULA PHYSEAL FRACTURES

(Dias and Tachdjian Classification)

VI.   JUVENILE TILLAUX

      ISOLATED FRACTURE OF THE LATERAL PART OF THE
         DISTAL TIBIA PHYSIS, A SALTER-HARRIS III FRACTURE

VI.

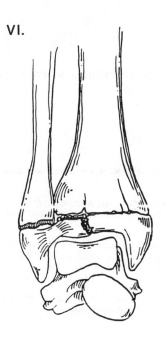

DISTAL TIBIA AND FIBULA PHYSEAL FRACTURES

(Dias and Tachdjian Classification)

VII. TRIPLANE

    FRACTURE PATTERN IN 3 PLANES WITH 3 FRAGMENTS.

    ONE FRAGMENT IS THE ANTEROLATERAL PORTION OF THE DISTAL TIBIA, A SALTER-HARRIS III FRACTURE

    THE SECOND FRAGMENT IS THE REMAINDER OF THE PHYSIS AND THE POSTERIOR SPIKE OF THE DISTAL TIBIA METAPHYSIS, A SALTER-HARRIS II FRACTURE

    THE THIRD FRAGMENT IS THE REMAINDER OF THE DISTAL TIBIAL METAPHYSIS AND SHAFT

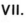

VII.

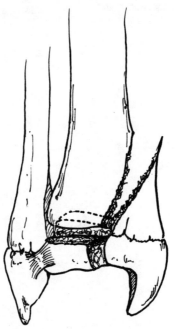

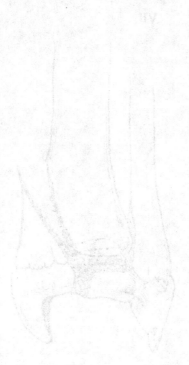

OSTEONECROSIS AND OSTEOCHONDROSIS

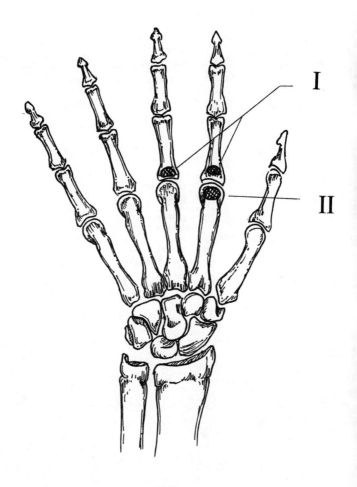

I

II

I.   SCAPHOID
     (PREISER)

II. LUNATE
     (KIENBÖCK)

III. DISTAL ULNA
     (BURNS)

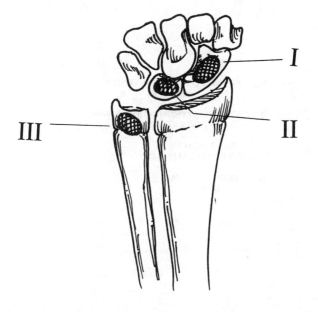

I.   PRIMORY OSSIFICATION CENTER
     (KÖHLER)

II. SECONDARY OSSIFICATION CENTER
     (SINDING-LARSEN)

III. TIBIA TUBERCLE
     (OSGOOD-SCHLATTER)

IV. MEDIAL PROXIMAL
     (BLOUNT)

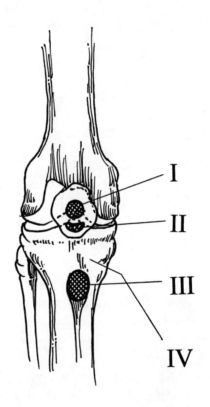

I. DISTAL TIBIA
    (LIFFERT-ARKIN)

II. TALUS
    (DIAZ)

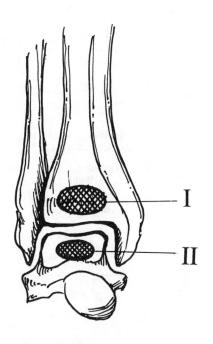

I

II

I. VERTEBRAL DISC
(SCHMORL-BEADLE)

II. VERTEBRAL BODY
(CALVÉ)

III. VERTEBRAL EPIPHYSIS
(SCHEUERMANN)

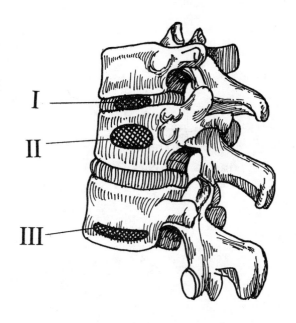

I.   FEMORAL EPIPHYSIS
       (LEGG- CALVÉ-PERTHES)

II.   GREATER TROCHANTER
        (MANDL)

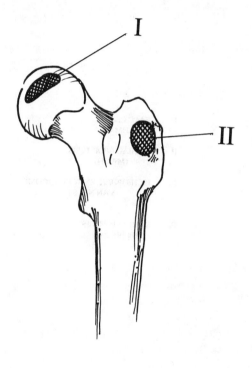

I. ILIAC CREST
(BUCHMAN)

II. ISCHIAL APOPHYSIS
(MILCH)

III. ISCHIOPUBIC SYNCHONDROSIS
(VAN NECK)

IV. SYMPYSIS PUBIS
(PIERSON)

214

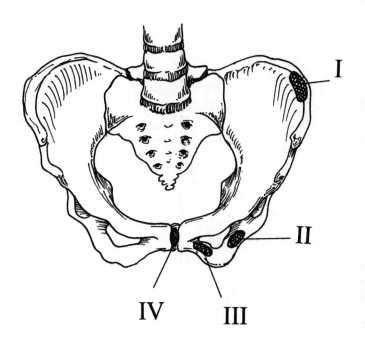

215

I.   NAVICULAR
        (KÖHLER)

II.   SECOND METATARSAL
        (FRIEBERG)

III.   FIFTH METATARSAL
        (ISELIN)

IV.   CALCANEUS APOPHYSIS
        (SEVER)

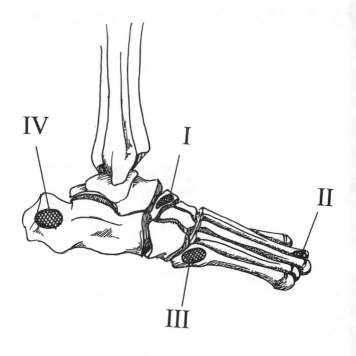

I.   HUMERAL HEAD
(HASS)

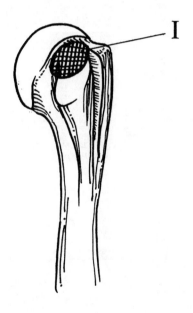

I.   **CAPITELLUM**
        (PANNER)

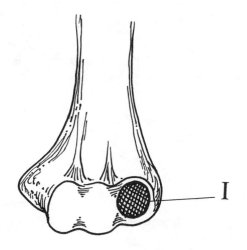

I

EPONYMS

AVIATOR'S ASTRAGALUS

Implies a variety of fractures of the talus; described after World War I as rudder bar is driven into foot during a plane crash.

BARTON'S FRACTURE

Displaced articular lip fracture of the distal radius; may be associated with carpal subluxation. Fracture configuration may be in a dorsal or volar direction.

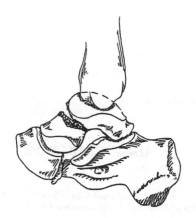

Aviator's Astragalus

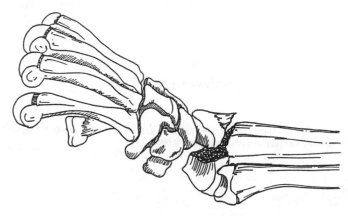

Barton's Fracture

BENNETT'S FRACTURE

Oblique fracture of the first metacarpal base separating a small triangular volar lip fragment from the proximally displaced metacarpal shaft.

BOSWORTH FRACTURE

Fracture of the distal fibula with fixed displacement of the proximal fragment posteriorly behind the posterolateral tibial ridge.

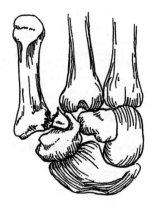

Bennett's Fracture

Bosworth Fracture

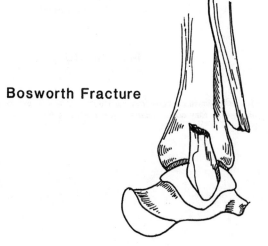

BOXER'S FRACTURE

Fracture of the fifth metacarpal neck with volar displacement of the metacarpal head.

BURST FRACTURE

Fracture of the vertebral body from axial load, usually with outward displacement of the fragments. May occur in cervical, thoracic, or lumbar spine.

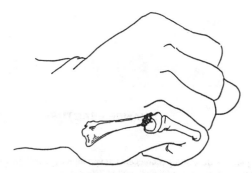

Boxer's Fracture

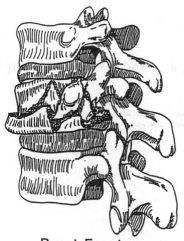

Burst Fracture

CHANCE FRACTURE

Distraction fracture of the thoracolumbar vertebral body with horizontal disruption of the spinous process, neural arch, and vertebral body.

CHAUFFEUR'S FRACTURE (HUTCHINSON'S FRACTURE)

Oblique fracture of the radial styloid, initially attributed to the starting crank of an engine being forcibly reversed by a backfire.

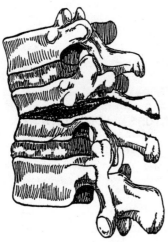

Chance Fracture

Chauffeur's Fracture

(Hutchinson's Fracture)

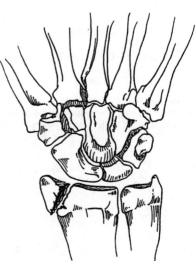

.RT'S FRACTURE and DISLOCATION

Fracture and/or dislocation involving Chopart's joints (talonavicular and calcaneocuboid joints) of the foot.

CLAY-SHOVELER'S (COAL-SHOVELER'S) FRACTURE

Spinous process fracture of the lower cervical or upper thoracic vertebrae. Injury initially attributed to workers attempting to throw upwards a full shovel of clay, but the clay adhered to the shovel causing a sudden flexion force opposite to the neck musculature.

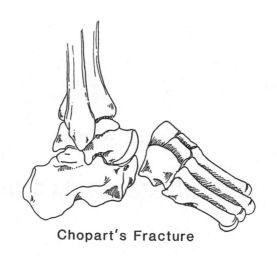

Chopart's Fracture

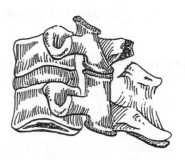

Clay Shoveler's (Coal Shoveler's)
Fracture

COLLES' FRACTURE

General term for fractures of the distal radius with dorsal displacement, with or without an ulnar styloid fracture. See Frykman's classification for further details.

COTTON'S FRACTURE

Trimalleolar ankle fracture with fractures of both malleoli and posterior lip of the tibia.

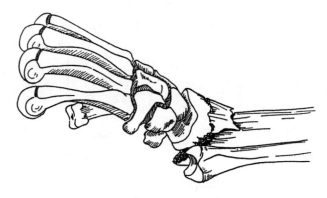

Colle's Fracture

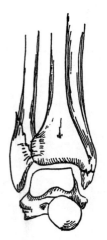
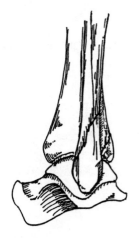

Cotton's Fracture

COZEN'S FRACTURE

Proximal tibia metaphyseal fracture that develops valgus deformity.

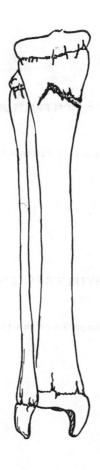

DIE PUNCH FRACTURE

Intra-articular distal radius fracture with impaction of the dorsal aspect of the lunate fossa.

DUPUYTREN'S FRACTURE

Fracture of the distal fibula with rupture of the distal tibiofibular ligaments and lateral displacement of the talus.

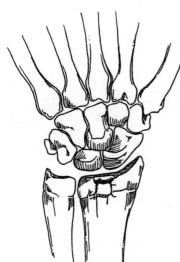

Die Punch Fracture

Dupuytren's Fracture

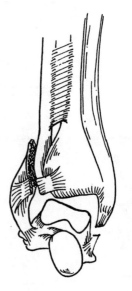

DUVERNEY'S FRACTURE

Fracture of the iliac wing without disruption of the pelvic ring.

ESSEX - LOPRESTI'S FRACTURE

Radial head fracture with associated dislocation of the distal radioulnar joint.

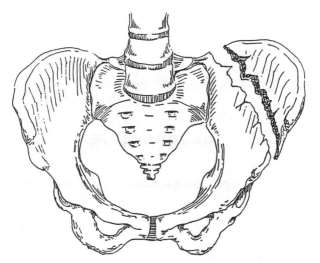

Duverney's Fracture

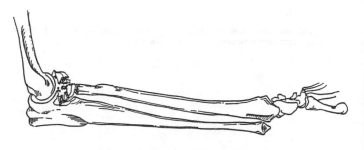

Essex-Lopresti's Fracture

GALEAZZI'S FRACTURE

Fracture of the radius in the distal third associated with subluxation of the distal ulna.

GREENSTICK FRACTURE

Incompletely fractured bone in a child, with a portion of the cortex and periosteum remaining intact on the compression side of the fracture.

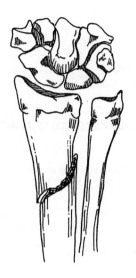

Galeazzi's Fracture

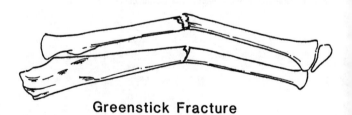

Greenstick Fracture

HAHN - STEINTHAL FRACTURE

Fracture of the capitellum involving a large osseous portion and may involve adjacent trochlea. See classification section for further details of capitellum fractures.

HANGMAN'S FRACTURE

Fracture through the neural arch of the second cervical vertebrae (axis).

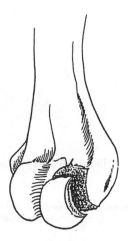

Hahn–Steinthal Fracture

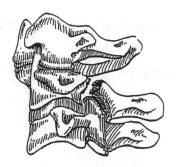

Hangman's Fracture

HILL - SACHS FRACTURE

Posterolateral humeral head compression fracture caused by anterior glenohumeral dislocation and impaction of the humeral head against the anterior glenoid rim.

HOLSTEIN - LEWIS FRACTURE

Fracture of the distal third of the humerus with entrapment of the radial nerve.

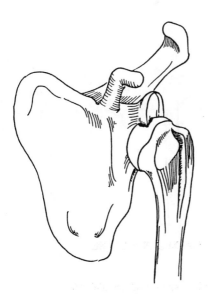

**Hill–Sachs
Fracture**

**Holstein–Lewis
Fracture**

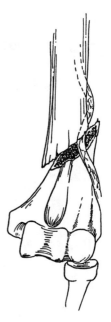

HUTCHISON'S FRACTURE

See CHAUFFEUR'S FRACTURE, pp 208 - 209.

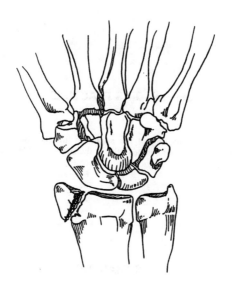

Hutchinson's Fracture

JEFFERSON'S FRACTURE

Comminuted fracture of the ring of the atlas due to axial compressive forces. Fractures usually occur anterior and posterior to the lateral facet joints.

JONES FRACTURE

Diaphyseal fracture of the base of the fifth metatarsal.

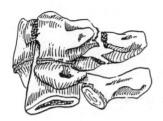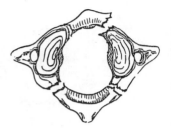

Jefferson's Fracture

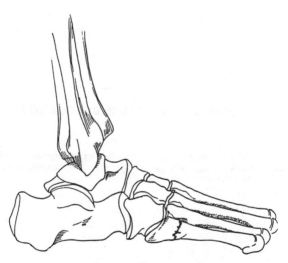

Jones Fracture

KOCHER - LORENZ FRACTURE

Slice fracture of the capitellum involving articular cartilage with minimal subchondral bone. See classification section for further details of capitellum fractures.

LISFRANC'S FRACTURE DISLOCATION

Fracture and/or dislocation involving Lisfranc's (tarsometatarsal) joint of the foot. Lisfranc was one of Napoleon's surgeons and described traumatic foot amputation through the tarsometatarsal joint level.

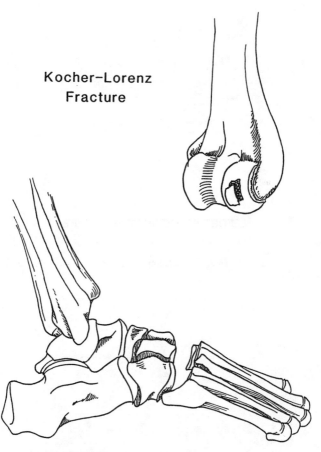

Kocher-Lorenz
Fracture

Lisfranc's Fracture Dislocation

LEFORT-WAGSTAFFE FRACTURE

Avulsion fracture of the anterior fibula tubercle caused by the anterior tibiofibular ligament.

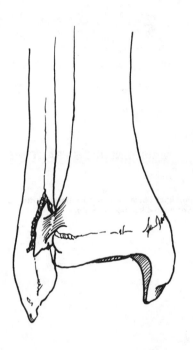

MAISONNEUVE'S FRACTURE

Fracture of the proximal fibula with syndesmosis rupture and associated medial malleolus fracture or deltoid ligament rupture.

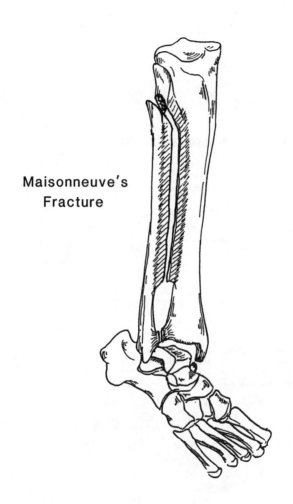

Maisonneuve's
Fracture

MALGAIGNE'S FRACTURE

Unstable pelvic fracture with vertical fractures anterior and posterior to the hip joint.

MALLET FINGER

Flexion deformity of the distal interphalangeal joint caused by extensor tendon separation from the distal phalanx. The deformity may be secondary to direct injury of the extensor tendon or an avulsion fracture from the dorsum of the distal phalanx where the tendon inserts.

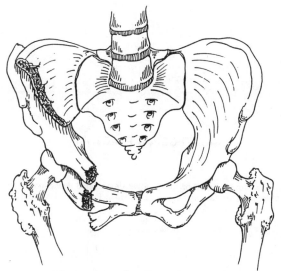

Malgaigne's Fracture

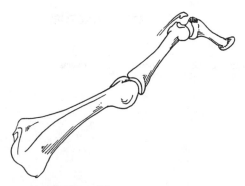

Mallet Finger

MONTEGGIA'S FRACTURE

Fracture of the proximal third of the ulna with associated dislocation of the radial head. Fracture complex has been further classified by Bado; see classification section.

NIGHTSTICK FRACTURE

Isolated fracture of the ulna secondary to direct trauma.

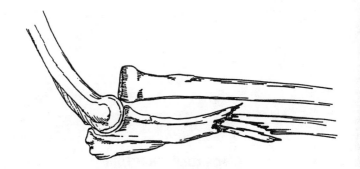

Monteggia's Fracture

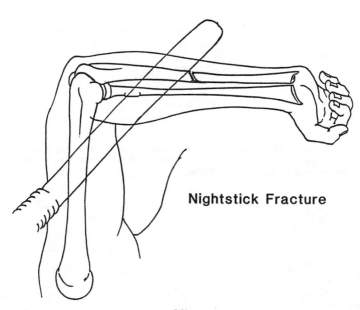

Nightstick Fracture

POSADAS' FRACTURE

Transcondylar humerus fracture with displacement of the distal fragment anteriorly and dislocation of the radius and ulna from the bicondylar fragment.

POTT'S FRACTURE

Fracture of the fibula within 2 to 3 inches above the lateral malleolus with rupture of the deltoid ligament and lateral subluxation of the talus. Pott did not describe disruption of the tibiofibular ligaments.

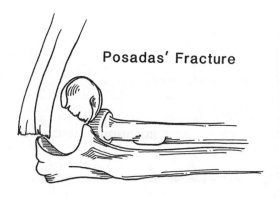

Posadas' Fracture

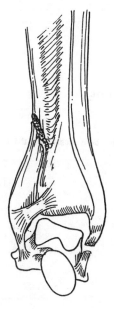

Pott's Fracture

ROLANDO'S FRACTURE

Y-shaped intra-articular fracture of the thumb metacarpal.

SEGOND'S FRACTURE

Avulsion fracture of the lateral tibial condyle from the bony insertion of the iliotibial band.

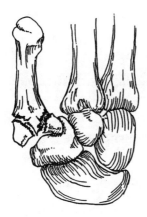

Rolando's Fracture

Segond's Fracture

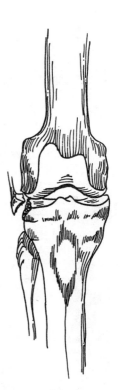

SHEPHERD'S FRACTURE

Fracture of the lateral tubercle of the posterior talar process.

SMITH'S FRACTURE

Fracture of the distal radius with palmar displacement of the distal fragment. Also referred to as a reverse Colles' fracture.

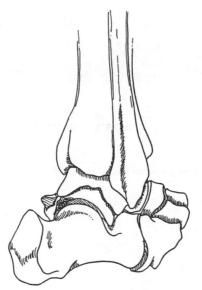

Shepherd's Fracture

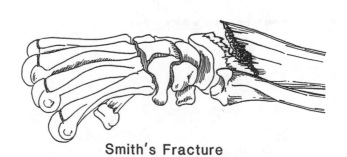

Smith's Fracture

STIEDA'S FRACTURE

Avulsion fracture of the medial femoral condyle at the origin of the medial collateral ligament.

STRADDLE FRACTURE

Bilateral fractures of the superior and inferior pubic rami.

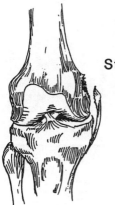

Stieda's Fracture

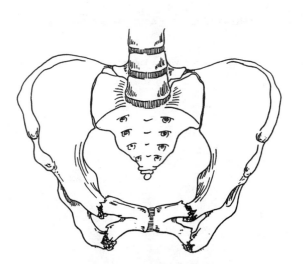

Straddle Fracture

THURSTON HOLLAND FRAGMENT

Metaphyseal fragment that occurs with a Salter-Harris II growth plate injury.

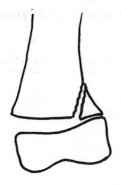

TEARDROP FRACTURE

Flexion fracture dislocation of the cervical spine with associated triangular anterior fragment of the involved vertebrae. Injury complex is unstable with posterior ligamentous disruption.

TILLAUX'S FRACTURE

Fracture of the lateral half of the distal tibial physis during differential closure of the physis. The medial part of the tibial physis has already fused.

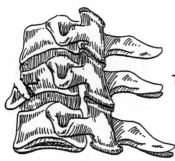

Teardrop Fracture

Tillaux's Fracture

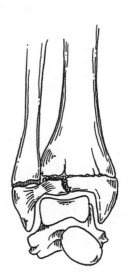

TILLAUX-CHAPUT FRACTURE

Avulsion fracture of the anterior lateral tibial margin caused by the anterior tibiofibular ligament.

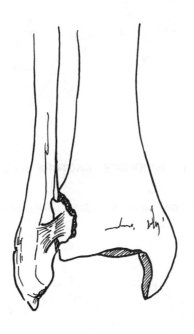

TODDLER'S FRACTURE

Spiral fracture of the tibia in infants and children, usually caused by low energy torsional forces.

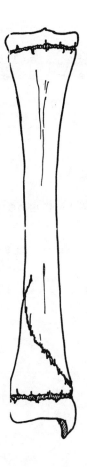

TRIPLANE FRACTURE

Fracture in 3 planes with 3 fragments.

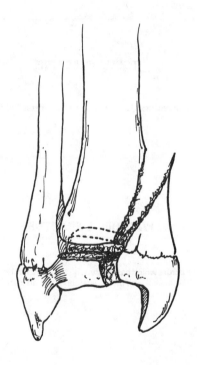

TORUS FRACTURE

Impaction fracture of childhood as the bone buckles instead of fracturing completely.

WALTHER'S FRACTURE

Ischioacetabular fracture which passes through the pubic rami and extends toward the sacroiliac joint. The medial wall of the acetabulum is displaced inward.

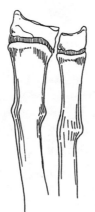

Torus Fracture

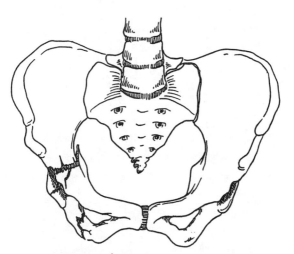

Walther's Fracture

REFERENCES

Anderson, H.G.: *The Medical and Surgical Aspects of Aviation*, Oxford University Press, London, 1919.

Anderson, L.D.: "Fractures of the Shafts of the Radius and Ulnar, In Rockwood, C.A., and D.P. Green (Eds.), *Fractures in Adults, Second Edition*, J.B. Lippincott, Philadelphia, 1983, pp. 511-558.

Anderson, L.D., and R.T. D'Alonzo: "Fractures of the Odontoid Process of the Axis," *J. Bone Joint Surg.* **46A**: 310-233, 1970.

Ashurst, A.P.C.: "An Anatomical and Surgical Study of Fractures of the Lower End of the Humerus," *The Samuel D. Gross Prize Essay of the Philadelphia Academy of Surgery, 1910*, Lea and Febiger, Philadelphia, 1910.

Bado, J.L.: "The Onteggia Lesion," *Clin. Orthoped.* **50**: 71-86, 1967.

Barton, J.R.: "Views and Treatment of an Important Injury to the Wrist," *Med. Examiner* 1: 365, 1838.

Baumann, J.U., and R.D. Campbell, Jr.: "Significance of Architectural Types of Fractures of the Carpal Scaphoid and Relation to Timing of Treatment," *J. Trauma* 2: 431-438, 1962.

Bennett, E.H.: "Fractures of the Metacarpal Bones," *Dublin J. Med. Sci.* **73**: 72-75, 1882.

Bosworth, D.M.: "Fracture Dislocation of the Ankle with Fixed Displacement of the Fibula Behind the Tibia," *J. Bone Joint Surg.* **29**: 130-135, 1947.

Brower, A.C.: *Orthopaedic Ranks North America* vol 14, No.19: pp332, 1983

Bryan, R.S.: "Fractures About the Elbow in Adults," *AAOS Instructional Course Lectures* **30**: 200-223, 1981.

Bryan, R.S., and B.F. Morrey: "Fractures of the Distal Humerus," In Morrey, B.F. (Ed.), *The Elbow and Its Disorders*, W.B. Saunders, Philadelphia, 1985, pp. 325-327.

Bucholz, R.W., K. and Gill: "Classification of Injuries of the Thoracolumbar Spine," *Orthoped. Clin. North. Am.* **17**: 67-73, 1986.

Cancelmo, Jr., J.J.: "Clay-Shoveler's Fracture. A Helpful Diagnostic Sign," *Am. J. Roentgenol.* **115**: 540, 1972.

Cass, J.R.: "Fractures and Dislocations Involving the Midfoot," In Chapman, M.W. (Ed.), *Operative Orthopaedics*. J.B. Lippincott, Philadelphia, 1988, pp. 1737-1755.

Chance, C.Q.: "Note on a Type of Flexion Fracture of the Spine," *Br. J. Radiol.* **21**: 452-453, 1948.

Chaput, V.: *Fractures Mallolaires du Cou-de-pied et les Accidents du Travail*, Paris, Masson and Cie, 1907.

Chapman, M.W. (Ed.): *Operative Orthopaedics*, J.B. Lippincott, Philadelphia, 1988.

Chutro, P.: *Fractures de la Extremidad Inferior Del Humero en los Ninos.* Theses J. Peuser, Buenos Airs, 1904.

Colles, A.: "On the Fracture of the Carpal Extremity of the Radius," *Edinburg. Med. Surg. J.* **10**: 182-186, 1814.

283

Colonna, P.C.: "Fractures of the Neck of the Femur in Childhood. A Report of Six Cases," *Ann. Surg.* **88**: 902, 1928.

Colton, C.L.: "Fractures of the Olecranon in Adults: Classification and Management," *Injury* **5**: 121-129, 1973-74.

Cotton, F.J.: "A New Type of Ankle Fracture," *J. Am. Med. Assoc.* **64**: 318-321, 1915.

Cozen, L.: "Fracture of the Proximal Portion of the Tibia in Children Followed by a Valgus Deformity," *Surg. Gynec. Obstet.* **97**: 183-188, 1953.

Dameron, T.B., and C.A. Rockwood: "Fractures and Dislocations of the Shoulder," In Rockwood, C.A., K.E. Wilkins, and R.E. K.E., King (Eds.), *Fractures in Children*, J.B. Lippincott, Philadelphia, 1984, pp. 624-653.

DeLee, J.S.: "Fractures and Dislocations of the Foot," In Mann, R.A. (Ed.), *Surgery of the Foot*, C.V. Mosby, St. Louis, 1986, pp. 592-714.

Denis, F.: "The Three Column Spine and Its Significance in the Classification of Acute Thoracolumbar Spinal Injuries," *Spine* **8**: 817-831, 1983.

Denis, F., S. Davis, and T. Comfort: "Sacral Fractures: An Important Problem," *Clin. Orthoped.* **227**: 67-81, 1988.

DePalma, A.F.: *The Management of Fractures and Dislocations*, W.B. Saunders, Philadelphia, 1959.

Destot, E.: *Injuries of the Wrist*, Ernest Benn, London, 1925.

Dias, L.S.: "Fractures of the Tibia and Fibula," In Rockwood, C.A., and D.P. Green, (Eds.), *Fractures in Children*, J.B. Lippincott, Philadelphia, 1984, pp. 983-1042.

Dias, L.S., and M.O. Tachdjian: "Physeal Injuries of the Ankle in Children," *Clin. Orthoped*, **136**: 230-233, 1978.

Dimon, J.H., and J.S. Hughston: "Unstable Intertrochanteric Fractures of the Hip," *J. Bone Joint Surg.* **49A**: 440-450, 1967.

Dunbar, J.S., H.F. Owen, M.B. Nogrady, and R. MeLesse: "Obscure Tibial Fracture of Infants - The Toddler's Fracture," *J. Can. Assoc. Radiol.* **25**: 136-144, 1964.

Dupuytren, G.: "Of Fractures of the Lower Extremity of the Fibula, and Luxations of the Foot," Reprinted In: *Medical Classics* **4**: 151-172, 1939.

Duverney, J.G.: *Traite des Maladies des Os*. Volume 1, DeBure L'Aine', 1751.

Edwards, H.C.: "Mechanism and Treatment of Backfire Fracture," *J. Bone Joint Surg.* **8**: 701-717, 1926.

Essex-Lopresti, P.: "Fractures of the Radial Head with Distal Radio-ulnar Dislocation. Report of Two Cases," *J. Bone Joint Surg.* **33B**: 224-247, 1951.

Essex-Lopresti, P.: "Results of Reduction in Fractures of the Calcaneum," *J. Bone Joint Surg.* **33B**: 284, 1951.

Essex-Lopresti, P.: "The Mechanism, Reduction Techniques, and Results in Fractures of the Os Calcis," *Br. J. Surg.* **39**: 395-419, 1952.

Fielding, J.W., and R.J. Hawkins: "Atlanto-axial Rotatory Fixation," *J. Bone Joint Surg.* **59A**: 37-44, 1977.

Frykman, G.: "Fractures of the Distal Radium Including Sequelae - Shoulder, Hand, Finger Syndrome, Disturbance in the Distal Radio-Ulnar Joint and Impairment of Nerve Functions," *Acta Orthoped. Scand.* **Suppl.** **108**: 1-153, 1967.

Galeazzi, R.: "Uber ein Besonderes Syndrom bei Verlrtzunger im Bereich der Unter Armknochen," *Arch. Orthop. Unfallchir.* **35**: 557-562, 1934.

Garden, R.S.: "Stability and Union in Subcapital Fractures of the Femur," *J. Bone Joint Surg.* **46B**: 630-647, 1964.

Green, D.P., and E.T. O'Brien: "Fractures of the Thumb Metacarpal," *Southern Med. J.* **65**: 807-814, 1972.

Green, D.P., and S.A. Rowland: "Fractures and Dislocations in the Hand," In Rockwood, C.A., D.P. Green (Eds.), *Fractures in Adults, Second Edition*, J.B. Lippincott, Philadelphia, 1984, pp. 313-410.

Gustilo, R.B., R.M. Mendoza, and D.N. Williams: "Problems in the Management of Type III (Severe) Open Fractures. A New Classification of Type III Open Fractures," *J. Trauma* **24**: 742-746, 1984.

Hahn, N.F.: "Fall von eine Besonderes Varietat der Frakturen des Ellenbogens," *Zeitschrift Qundarzte und Geburtshelte* **6**: 185-189, 1853.

Harris, J.H., B. Edeiken-Monroe, and D.R. Kopaniky: "A Practical Classification of Acute Cervical Spine Injuries," *Orthoped. Clin. North Am.* **17**: 15-30, 1986.

Hawkins, L.G.: "Fractures of the Neck of the Talus," *J. Bone Joint Surg.* **47A**: 1170-1175, 1965.

Heckman, J.D.: "Fractures and Dislocations of the Foot," In Rockwood, C.A., and D.P. Green (Eds.), *Fractures in Adults, Second Edition*, J.B. Lippincott, Philadelphia, 1984, pp. 1703-1832.

Hill, H.A., and M.D. Sachs: "The Grooved Defect of the Humeral Head. A Frequently Unrecognized Complication of Dislocations of the Shoulder Joint," *Radiology* **35**: 690-700, 1940.

Holland, C.T.: "A Radiographic Note on Injuries to the Distal Epiphysis of the Radius and Ulna," *Proc. Royal Soc. Med.* **22**: 695-700, 1929.

Holstein, A., G.B. Lewis: "Fractures of the Humerus with Radial Nerve Paralysis," *J. Bone Joint Surg.* **45A**: 1382, 1963.

Holdsworth, F.W.: "Fractures, Dislocations, and Fracture-dislocations of the Spine," *J. Bone Joint Surg.* **45B**: 6-20, 1963.

Hoppenfield, S., P. deBoer: *Surgical Exposures in Orthopaedics. The Anatomic Approach*, J.B. Lippincott, Philadelphia, 1984, p. 507.

Ideberg, R.: "Fractures of the Scapula Involving the Glenoid Fossa," In Bateman, J.E., and R.P. Welsh (Eds.), *Surgery of the Shoulder*, B.C. Becker, New York, 1984, pp. 63-66.

Jefferson, G.: "Fracture of Atlas Vertebrae: Report of Four Cases, and a Review of Those Previously Recorded," *Br. J. Surg.* **7**: 407-422, 1920.

Johnston, G.W.: "A Follow-up of One Hundred Cases of Fracture of the Head of the Radius with a Review of the Literature," *Ulster Med. J.* **31**: 51-56, 1962.

Jones, R.: "Fracture of the Base of the Fifth Metatarsal Bone by Indirect Violence," *Ann. Surg.* **35**: 697-700, 1902.

Kaplan, L.: "The Treatment of Fractures and Dislocations of the Hand and Fingers. Technic of Unpadded Casts for Carpal, Metacarpal and Phalangeal Fractures," *Surg. Clin. North Am.* **20**: 1695-1720, 1940.

Kocher, T.: *Beitrage zur Kenntniss Einiger Tisch Wichtiger Frakturforman*, Sallman, Basel, 1896, pp. 585-591.

Kyle, R.F., R.B. Gustilo, and R.F. Premer: "Analysis of 622 Intertrochanteric Hip Fractures: A Retrospective and Prospective Study," *J. Bone Joint Surg.* **61A**: 216-221, 1979.

Lauge-Hansen, N.: "Ligamentous Ankle Fractures: Diagnosis and Treatment," *Acta. Chir. Scan.* **97**: 544-550, 1949.

LeFort, L.: "Note sur une Variete non Decrete de Fracture Verticale de la Malleole Esterne par Arrachement," *Bull. Gen. Ther.* **110**: 193-199, 1886.

Lorenz, H.: "Zur Kenntniss der Fraktura Humeri (Eminentiae Capitate)," *Deutsche Zeitschr. f. Chir.* **78**: 531-545, 1905.

Maisonneuve, J.B.: "Recherches sur la Fracture du Perone," *Arch. Gen. Med.* **7**: 165-187, 433-473, 1840.

Malgaigne, J.F.: *Treatise on Fractures*, J.B. Lippincott, Philadelphia, 1959.

Mason, J.A., and N.M. Shutkin: "Immediate Active Motion Treatment of Fractures of the Head and Neck of the Radius," *Surg. Gynecol. Obstet.* **76**: 731-737, 1943.

Meyers, M.H., and F.M. McKeever: "Fractures of the Intercondylar Eminence of the Tibia," *J. Bone Joint Surg.* **52A**: 1677-1684, 1970.

Milch, H.: "Fractures and Fracture Dislocations of the Humeral Condyles," *J. Trauma* **4**: 592-607, 1964.

Monteggia, G.B.: *Instituzioni Chirrugiche, Volume 5*, Maspero, Milan, 1814.

Morrey, B.F.: *The Elbow and Its Disorder*, W.B. Saunders, Philadelphia, 1985.

Muller, M.E., M. Allgower, R. Schneider, and H. Willenegger: *Manual of Internal Fixation, Second Edition*, Springer-Verlag, New York, 1979.

Neer, C.S., II: "Displaced Proximal Humeral Fractures: I. Classification and Evaluations," *J. Bone Joint Surg.* **52A**: 1077-1089, 1970.

Neer, C.S., II: "Fractures of the Distal Third of the Clavicle," *Clin. Orthoped.* **58**: 43-50, 1968.

Ogden, J.A.: "The Uniqueness of Growing Bones," In Rockwood, C.A., K.E. Wilkens, and R.E. King (Eds.), *Fractures in Children*, J.B. Lippincott, Philadelphia, 1984, pp. 1-86.

Pantazopoulus, T., P. Galanos, P., E. Voganas, *et al.*: "Fractures of the Neck of the Talus," *Acta. Orthoped. Scand.* **45**: 296-306, 1974.

Pipkin, G.: "Treatment of Grade IV Fracture-Dislocation of the Hip," *J. Bone Joint Surg.* **39A**: 1027-1042, 1957.

Pirone, A.M., H.K. Graham, and J.I. Krajbich: "Management of Displaced Extension-type Supracondylar Fractures of the Humerus in Children," *J. Bone Joint Surg.* **70A**: 641-650, 1988.

Pott, P.: *Some Few General Remarks on Fractures and Dislocations*, Hawes, Clarks, Collins, London, 1768.

Quenu, E. and G. Kuss: "Etude sur les Luxations du Metatarse (Luxations Metatarso-Transiennes) due Diastasis entre le I. et le Metatarsien," *Rev. Chir. (Paris)*, **39**: 281-336, 720-791, 1093-1134, 1909.

Rang, M.: *The Growth Plate and Its Disorders*, Williamsand Wilkins, Baltimore, 1969.

Regan, W., and B. Morrey: "Fractures of the Coronoid Process of the Ulna," *J. Bone Joint Surg.* **71A**: 1348-1354, 1989.

Resnick, D., and Niwayama, G.: *Diagnosis of Bone and Joint Disorders, Second Edition*, W.B. Saunders, Phiadelphia, 1988 Chapters 82 & 84

Riseborough, E.J., and E.L. Radin: "Intercondylar T Fractures of the Humerus in the Adult," *J. Bone Joint Surg.* **51A**: 130-141, 1969.

Roberts, J.B., and J.A. Kelly: *Treatise on Fractures, Second Edition*, J.B. Lippincott, Philadelphia, 1921.

Rockwood Jr., C.A., and D.P. Green (Eds.): *Fractures in Adults, Second Edition*, J.B. Lippincott, Philadelphia, 1984.

Rolando, S.: "Fracture de la Base du Premier Metcarpien: Et Principalement sur une Variete non Encore Decrits," *Presse Med.* 33: 303, 1910.

Ruedi, T., and M. Allgower: "Fractures of the Lower End of the Tibia into the Ankle Joint," *Injury* 1: 92, 1969.

Russe, O.: "Fracture of the Carpal Navicular: Diagnosis, Non-operative Treatment, and Operative Treatment," *J. Bone Joint Surg.* 42A: 759-768, 1960.

Salter, R.B., and W.R. Harris: "Injuries Involving the Epiphyseal Plate," *J. Bone Joint Surg.* 45A: 587-622, 1963.

Schatzker, J.: "Compression in the Surgical Treatment of Fractures of the Tibia," *Clin. Orthoped.* 105: 220-239, 1974.

Scheck, M." "Long Term Follow Up of Treatment of Comminuted Fractures of the Distal End of the Radius by Transfixion with Kirschner Wires and Case," *J. Bone Joint Surg.* 44A: 337-351, 1962.

Schneider, R.C., and E.A. Kahn: "Chronic Neurological Sequelae of Acute Trauma to the Spine and Spinal Cord. Part I. The Significance of the Acute Flexion or "Teardrop" Fracture-dislocation of the Cervical Spine," *J. Bone Joint Surg.* 38A: 985-997, 1956.

Segond, P.: "Rechershes Cliniques et Experimentaelis sur les Epanchements Sanquins du Genou par Entorse," *Prog. Met. (Paris)* 7: 297, 1879.

Seinsheimer, F.: "Subtrochanteric Fractures of the Femur. *J. Bone Joint Surg.* 60A: 300-306, 1978.

Shepherd, F.J.: "A Hitherto Undescribed Fracture of the Astragalus," *J. Anat. Physiol.* 18: 79-81, 1882.

Smith R.W.: *A Treatise on Fractures in the Vicinity of Joints, and on Certain Forms of Accidental and Congenital Dislocation*, Hodges and Smith, Dublin, 1854.

Stark, H.H., J.H. Bayes, and J.N. Wilson: "Mallet Finger," *J. Bone Joint Surg.* 44A: 1061-1068, 1962.

Steinthal, D.: "Die Isolierte Fraktur der Eminentia Capitat in Ellenbogengelenk," *Centrallbl. f. Chirugi* 15: 17-20, 1898.

Stieda, A.: *Arch. f. Klin. Chir.* 85: 815, 1908.

Tillaux, P.: *Traite de Chirurgie Clinique*, Vol. 2, Paris, Asselin & Houzeau, 1848.

Tile, M.: "Pelvic Ring Fractures: Should They be Fixed," *J. Bone Joint Surg.* 70B: 1-12, 1988.

Tile, M.: *Fractures of the Pelvis and Acetabulum*, Williams and Wilkins, Baltimore, 1984.

Wagstaffe, W.W.: "An Unusual Form of Fracture of the Fibular," *Saint Thomas Hospital Reports* 6: 43, 1875.

Walther, C.: "Recherches Experimentelles sur Certains Fracturas de la Cavietecotyloide," *Bull. Soc. Anat. Paris* 5: 561, 1891.

Watson-Jones, R.: *Fractures and Joint Injuries, Volume 2, 3rd Edition*, Williams and Wilkins, Baltimore, 1946.

Wilkins, K.E.: "Fractures and Dislocations of the Elbow Region," In Rockwood, C.A., K.E. Wilkins, and R.E. King (Eds.), *Fractures in Children, Third Edition*, J.B. Lippincott, Philadelphia, pp. 509-828, 1991.

Winquist, R.A., S.T. Hansen, Jr., and D.K. Clawson: "Closed Intramedullary Nailing of Femoral Fractures: A Report of Five Hundred and Twenty Cases," *J. Bone Joint Surg.* **66A**: 529-539, 1984.

Wood-Jones, F.: "The Examination of Bodies of 100 Men Executed in Nubia in Roman Times," *Br. Med. J.* 1: 736-737, 1908.

Wood-Jones, F.: "The Ideal Lesion Produced by Judicial Hanging," *Lancet* 1: 53, 1913.

SELECTED

INDIVIDUAL

DRUG

PREPARATIONS

C-II: Controlled Substance, Schedule II
C-III: Controlled Substance, Schedule III
C-IV: Controlled Substance, Schedule IV
C-V: Controlled Substance, Schedule V

GENERIC NAME	COMMON TRADE NAMES	THERAPEUTIC CATEGORY	PREPARATIONS	COMMON ADULT DOSAGE
Acetaminophen (*)	ANACIN, ASPIRIN FREE	Non-Opioid Analgesic, Antipyretic	**Cplt, Tab & Gelcap: 500 mg**	1000 mg tid or qid po.
	PANADOL, MAXIMUM STRENGTH		**Cplt & Tab: 500 mg**	1000 mg q 4 h po.
	TYLENOL, REGULAR STRENGTH		**Cplt & Tab: 325 mg**	325 - 650 mg tid or qid po.
	TYLENOL, EXTRA-STRENGTH		**Cplt, Tab, Gelcap & Geltab: 500 mg**	1000 mg tid or qid po.
			Liquid: 500 mg/15 mL (7% alcohol)	30 mL (1000 mg) q 4 - 6 h po.
	TYLENOL SORE THROAT ADULT LIQUID		**Liquid: 500 mg/15 mL**	30 mL (1000 mg) q 4 - 6 h po.
	TYLENOL ARTHRITIS EXTENDED RELIEF		**Extended-Rel. Cplt: 650 mg**	1300 mg q 8 h po.
	FEVERALL, JUNIOR STRENGTH		**Rectal Suppos: 325 mg**	Insert 2 rectally q 4 - 6 h.
	ACETAMINOPHEN UNISERTS		**Rectal Suppos: 650 mg**	Insert 1 rectally q 4 - 6 h.
Acetylsalicylic Acid [see Aspirin]				
Alatrofloxacin Mesylate [see Trovafloxacin Mesylate (TROVAN)]				
Alendronate Sodium	FOSAMAX	Bone Stabilizer	**Tab: 5, 10, 35, 70, 40 mg**	Take at least 30 min. before the first food, beverage, or medication of the day. **Osteoporosis in Postmenopausal Women: Treatment:** 10 mg once daily po or 70 mg once weekly po. **Prevention:** 5 mg once daily po or 35 mg once weekly po. **Osteoporosis in Men:** 10 mg once daily po. **Glucocorticoid-Induced Osteoporosis:** 5 mg once daily po. For postmenopausal women

Alfentanil Hydrochloride (*) (C-II)	ALFENTA	Opioid Analgesic	Inj: 500 µg/mL	**Duration of Anesthesia:** **Under 30 min:** 8 - 20 µg/kg IV, followed by increments of 3 - 5 µg/kg IV q 5 - 20 minutes or 0.5 - 1 µg/kg/min IV. **30 - 60 min:** 20 - 50 µg/kg IV, followed by increments of 5 - 15 µg/kg IV q 5 - 20 minutes.
Amcinonide	CYCLOCORT	Corticosteroid	**Cream & Oint:** 0.1% **Lotion:** 0.1%	Apply to affected areas bid to tid. Rub into affected areas bid.
Amikacin Sulfate (*)	AMIKIN	Antibacterial	**Inj (per mL):** 50, 250 mg	**Usual Dosage:** 15 mg/kg/day IM or by IV infusion (over 30 - 60 min) divided in 2 or 3 equal doses at equal intervals. **Uncomplicated UTI:** 250 mg bid IM or by IV infusion (over 30 - 60 min).
Amoxicillin (*)	AMOXIL	Antibacterial	**Cpsl:** 250, 500 mg **Tab:** 500, 875 mg **Chewable Tab:** 125, 200, 250 mg **Powd for Susp (per 5 mL):** 125, 200, 250, 400 mg	Infections of the Lower Respiratory Tract 500 mg q 8 h po or 875 mg q 12 h po. **Gonorrheal Infections, Acute Uncomplicated:** 3 g (+ 1 g of probenecid) as a single po dose. **Other Susceptible Infections:** **Mild to Moderate:** 250 mg q 8 h po or 500 mg q 12 h po. **Severe:** 500 mg q 8 h po or 875 mg q 12 h po.
	WYMOX		**Cpsl:** 250, 500 mg **Powd for Susp (per 5 mL):** 125, 250 mg	Same dosages as for AMOXIL above.

not receiving estrogen - 10 mg once daily po.
Paget's Disease: 40 mg once daily po for 6 months.

GENERIC NAME	COMMON TRADE NAMES	THERAPEUTIC CATEGORY	PREPARATIONS	COMMON ADULT DOSAGE
Ampicillin Anhydrous (*)	OMNIPEN	Antibacterial	Cpsl: 250, 500 mg Powd for Susp (per 5 mL): 125, 250 mg	**Respiratory Tract and Soft Tissue Infections:** 250 mg q 6 h po. **Genitourinary or Gastrointestinal Tract Infect. other than Gonorrhea:** 500 mg q 6 h po. **Gonorrhea:** 3.5 g (plus 1.0 g of probenecid) as a single po dose.
Ampicillin Sodium (*)	OMNIPEN-N	Antibacterial	Powd for Inj: 125, 250, 500 mg; 1, 2 g	**Respiratory Tract and Soft Tissue Infections:** Under 40 kg: 25 - 50 mg/kg/day in equally divided doses at 6 - 8 h intervals IM or IV. Over 40 kg: 250 - 500 mg q 6 h IM or IV. **Genitourinary or Gastrointestinal Tract Infections Including Gonorrhea in Females:** Under 40 kg: 50 mg/kg/day in equally divided doses at 6 - 8 h intervals IM or IV. Over 40 kg: 500 mg q 6 h IM or IV. **Urethritis in Males due to N. gonorrhoeae:** Two doses of 500 mg each IM or IV at an interval of 8 - 12 h. Repeat if necessary. **Bacterial Meningitis:** 150 - 200 mg/kg/day in equally divided doses q 3 - 4 h. Treatment may be initiated with IV drip and continued with IM injections. **Septicemia:** 150 - 200 mg/kg/day. Start with IV administration for at least 3 days and continue with IM injections q 3 - 4 h.
Ampicillin Trihydrate (*)	PRINCIPEN	Antibacterial	Cpsl: 250, 500 mg Powd for Susp (per 5 mL): 125, 250 mg	Same dosages as for OMNIPEN above.
Aspirin (*)	BAYER CHILDREN'S ASPIRIN ASPIRIN REGIMEN BAYER	Non-Opioid Analgesic, Antipyretic, Antiinflammatory	Chewable Tab: 81 mg Enteric Coated Tab: 81 mg Enteric Coated Cplt: 325 mg	**Usual Dosage:** 325 - 650 mg q 4 h po. prn. **Analgesic or Antiinflammatory:** the OTC maximum dosage is 4000 mg per day po in divided doses.
Aspirin (*) [Continued]	BAYER ASPIRIN	Drug for Suspected Acute MI	Cplt, Gelcap & Tab: 325 mg	**Transient Ischemic Attacks in Men:** 1300 mg daily po in divided doses (650 mg bid or 325

BAYER ASPIRIN, EXTRA STRENGTH		Cplt, Gelcap & Tab: 500 mg	mg qid). **Suspected Acute Myocardial Infarction:** 160 to 162.5 mg po, as soon as the infarct is suspected & then daily for at least 30 days.
BAYER 8-HOUR ASPIRIN		Cplt: 650 mg	
ST. JOSEPH ADULT CHEWABLE ASPIRIN		Chewable Cplt: 81 mg	
ECOTRIN	Non-Opioid Analgesic, Antiinflammatory	Enteric Coated Tab: 81, 325, 500 mg	Same dosages as for ASPIRIN REGIMEN BAYER above.
ECOTRIN, BAYER ASPIRIN EXTRA-STRENGTH ARTHRITIS PAIN FORMULA	Non-Opioid Analgesic, Antiinflammatory	Enteric Coated Cplt: 500 mg	Same dosages as for ASPIRIN REGIMEN BAYER above.
EASPRIN	Non-Opioid Analgesic, Antiinflammatory	Enteric Coated Tab: 975 mg	1 tab tid to qid po.
HALFPRIN	Drug for Suspected Acute MI	Tab: 162 mg	162 mg po, taken as soon as the first infarct is suspected & then daily for at least 30 days.
Azithromycin Dihydrate (*) ZITHROMAX	Antibacterial	Cplt: 250 mg Tab: 250, 600 mg Powd for Susp (per 5 mL): 100, 200 mg Powd for Susp: 1 g packets	**Usual Dosage:** 500 mg po as a single dose on the first day followed by 250 mg once daily on days 2 through 5. Administer Suspension on an empty stomach; tablets may be taken with or without food. **Non-gonococcal Urethritis and Cervicitis due to *C. trachomatis*:** 1 g po as a single dose. Administer Suspension on an empty stomach; tablets may be taken with or without food. **Gonococcal Urethritis and Cervicitis due to *N. gonorrhea*:** 2 g po as a single dose. **Genital Ulcer Disease due to *H. ducrey*** (Chancroid): 1 g po as a single dose. **Prevention of Disseminated *Mycobacterium avium* Complex (MAC):** 1200 mg po once weekly.

293

GENERIC NAME	COMMON TRADE NAMES	THERAPEUTIC CATEGORY	PREPARATIONS	COMMON ADULT DOSAGE
Aztreonam (*)	AZACTAM	Antibacterial	**Powd for Inj:** 0.5, 1, 2 g **Inj (per 100 mL):** 0.5, 1, 2 g	**Urinary Tract Infections:** 0.5 - 1.0 g q 8 or 12 h by IV infusion or IM. **Moderately Severe Systemic Infections:** 1 - 2 g q 8 or 12 h by IV infusion. **Severe Systemic or Life-Threatening Infections:** 2 g q 6 or 8 h by IV infusion.
Bacampicillin Hydrochloride (*)	SPECTROBID	Antibacterial	**Tab:** 400 mg	**Upper Respiratory Tract Infections, Urinary Tract Infections, Skin and Skin Structure Infections:** 400 mg q 12 h po. **Lower Respiratory Tract Infections and Severe Infections:** 800 mg q 12 h po. **Gonorrhea, Acute Uncomplicated:** 1.6 g (plus 1 g of probenecid) as a single dose po.
Baclofen (*)	LIORESAL	Skeletal Muscle Relaxant	**Tab:** 10, 20 mg	5 mg tid po for 3 days; increase by 5 mg tid every 3 days (maximum 80 mg daily (20 mg qid)) until optimum effect is achieved.
Buprenorphine Hydrochloride (*) (C-V)	BUPRENEX	Opioid Analgesic	**Inj:** 0.3 mg/mL	0.3 mg by deep IM or slow IV (over at least 2 minutes) at up to 6-hour intervals. Repeat once, if required, in 30 - 60 minutes.
Butorphanol Tartrate (*) (C-IV)	STADOL STADOL NS	Opioid Analgesic	**Inj (per mL):** 1, 2 mg **Nasal Spray:** 10 mg/mL	**IM:** 2 mg. May be repeated q 3 - 4 h prn. **IV:** 1 mg. May be repeated q 3 - 4 h prn. 1 spray in one nostril. If pain is not relieved in 60 - 90 minutes, an additional 1 spray may be given. The initial 2 dose sequence may be repeated in 3 - 4 h prn.
Calcifediol	CALDEROL	Vitamin D Analog	**Cpsl:** 20, 50 µg	300 - 350 µg weekly po, administered on a daily or alternate-day schedule. Most patients respond to doses of 50 - 100 µg daily or 100 - 200 µg on alternate days.

Calcitriol (*)	ROCALTROL	Vitamin D Analog	**Cpsl:** 0.25, 0.5 µg **Solution:** 1.0 µg/mL	**Dialysis Patients:** 0.25 µg daily po. Dosage may be increased by 0.25 µg per day at 4 to 8 week intervals. Most patients respond to doses between 0.5 and 1 µg daily. **Predialysis Patients:** 0.25 µg daily po. Dosage may be increased to 0.5 µg daily if needed. **Hypoparathyroidism:** 0.25 µg daily po given in the AM. The dosage may be increased at 2 to 4 week intervals. Most patients respond to doses between 0.5 and 2 µg daily.
Calcium Carbonate (*)	CALTRATE 600	Calcium Supplement	**Tab:** 600 mg (as calcium)	1 or 2 tab daily po.
	OS-CAL 500	Calcium Supplement	**Tab:** 500 mg (as calcium)	500 mg bid or tid po with meals.
	TUMS	Calcium Supplement, Antacid	**Chewable Tab:** 500 mg	**Calcium Supplement:** Chew 2 tablets bid. **Antacid:** Chew 2 - 4 tablets q h prn. Do not take more than 16 tablets in 24 h.
	TUMS E-X		**Chewable Tab:** 750 mg	**Calcium Supplement:** Chew 2 tablets bid. **Antacid:** Chew 2 - 4 tablets q h prn. Do not take more than 10 tablets in 24 h.
	TUMS ULTRA		**Chewable Tab:** 1000 mg	**Calcium Supplement:** Chew 2 tablets bid. **Antacid:** Chew 2 - 3 tablets q h prn. Do not take more than 8 tablets in 24 h.
	TITRALAC TITRALAC EXTRA STRENGTH	Antacid	**Chewable Tab:** 420 mg **Cheable Tab:** 750 mg	Chew 2 tab q 2 - 3 h. Chew 1 - 2 tab q 2 - 3 h.
	ROLAIDS, CALCIUM RICH/ SODIUM FREE	Antacid	**Chewable Tab:** 550 mg	Chew 1 or 2 tab prn, up to a maximum of 14 tab per day.
	MYLANTA SOOTHING LOZENGES	Antacid	**Lozenges:** 600 mg	Allow 1 lozenge to dissolve in the mouth. If necessary, follow with a second. Repeat prn, up to 12 lozenges per day.

GENERIC NAME	COMMON TRADE NAMES	THERAPEUTIC CATEGORY	PREPARATIONS	COMMON ADULT DOSAGE
	ALKA-MINTS	Antacid	**Chewable Tab:** 850 mg	Chew 1 or 2 tablets q 2 h.
	MAALOX CAPLETS	Antacid	**Cplt:** 1000 mg	1000 mg po prn. Do not take more than 8 caplets in 24 h.
Carbenicillin Indanyl Sodium	GEOCILLIN	Antibacterial	**Tab:** 382 mg	**Urinary Tract Infections:** *E. coli, Proteus species,* and *Enterobacter.* 382 - 764 mg qid po. *Pseudomonas and Enterococcus:* 764 mg qid po. **Prostatitis:** 764 mg qid po.
Carisoprodol (*)	SOMA	Skeletal Muscle Relaxant	**Tab:** 350 mg	350 mg tid and hs po.
Cefaclor (*)	CECLOR	Antibacterial	**Powd for Susp (per 5 mL):** 125, 187, 250, 375 mg **Cpsl:** 250, 500 mg	**Usual Dosage:** 250 mg q 8 h po. For more severe infections or those caused by less susceptible organisms, the dosage may be doubled. **Secondary Bacterial Infections of Acute Bronchitis or Acute Bacterial Exacerabations of Chronic Bronchitis:** 500 mg q 12 h po for 7 days. **Pharyngitis or Tonsillitis:** 375 mg q 12 h po for 10 days. **Skin and Skin Structure Infections, Uncompl.:** 375 mg q 12 h po for 7 to 10 days.
	CECLOR CD		**Extended-Rel. Tab:** 375, 500 mg	375 - 500 mg q 12 h po for 7 - 10 days.
Cefadroxil Monohydrate (*)	DURICEF	Antibacterial	**Powd for Susp (per 5 mL):** 125, 250, 500 mg **Cpsl:** 500 mg **Tab:** 1 g	**Urinary Tract Infections:** **Lower, Uncomplicated:** 1 - 2 g daily po in single or divided doses (bid). **Other:** 2 g daily po in divided doses (bid). **Skin and Skin Structure Infections:** 1 g daily po in single or divided doses (bid). **Pharyngitis and Tonsillitis:** 1 g daily po in single or divided doses (bid) for 10 days.

Cefazolin Sodium (*)	ANCEF KEFZOL	Antibacterial	Powd for Inj: 500 mg, 1 g	**Moderate to Severe Infections:** 500 mg - 1 g q 6 - 8 h IM or IV. **Mild Infections caused by susceptible Gram Positive Cocci:** 250 - 500 mg q 8 h IM or IV. **Urinary Tract Infect, Acute, Uncomplicated:** 1 g q 12 h IM or IV. **Pneumococcal Pneumonia:** 500 mg q 12 h IM or IV. **Severe, Life-Threatening Infections (e.g., Septicemia):** 1 - 1.5 g q 6 h IM or IV.
Cefdinir (*)	OMNICEF	Antibacterial	Cpsl: 300 mg	**Community-Acquired Pneumonia and Skin and Skin Structure Infections, Uncomplicated:** 300 mg q 12 h po for 10 days. **Acute Exacerbations of Chronic Bronchitis & Acute Maxillary Sinusitis:** 300 mg q 12 h po or 600 mg q 24 h po for 10 days. **Pharyngitis / Tonsillitis:** 300 mg q 12 h po for 5 - 10 days or 600 mg q 24 h po for 10 days.
Cefditoren Pivoxil	SPECTRACEF	Antibacterial	Tab: 200 mg	**Acute Bacterial Exacerbation of Chronic Bronchitis:** 400 mg bid po for 10 days. **Pharyngitis/Tonsillitis and Skin & Skin Structure Infections (Uncomplicated):** 200 mg bid po for 10 days.
Cefepime Hydrochloride (*)	MAXIPIME	Antibacterial	Powd for Inj: 0.5, 1, 2 g	**Urinary Tract Infections:** **Mild to Moderate:** 0.5 - 1 g IM or IV (over 30 min.) q 12 h for 7 - 10 days. **Severe:** 2 g IV (over 30 min.) q 12 h for 10 days. **Pneumonia:** 1 - 2 g IV (over 30 min.) q 12 h for 10 days. **Skin & Skin Structure Infections:** 2 g IV (over 30 min.) q 12 h for 10 days. **Empiric Therapy for Febrile Neutropenic**
Cefixime (*)	SUPRAX	Antibacterial	Tab: 200, 400 mg	**Usual Dosage:** 400 mg once daily or 200 mg

GENERIC NAME	COMMON TRADE NAMES	THERAPEUTIC CATEGORY	PREPARATIONS	COMMON ADULT DOSAGE
			Powd for Susp: 100 mg/5 mL	q 12 h po. Gonorrhea, Uncomplicated: 400 mg once daily po.
Cefonicid Sodium (*)	MONOCID	Antibacterial	Powd for Inj: 0.5, 1 g	Usual Dosage: 1 g daily IV or deep IM. Urinary Tract Infections: 0.5 g q 24 h IV or deep IM. Mild to Moderate Infections: 1 g q 24 h IV or deep IM. Severe or Life-Threatening Infections: 2 g q 24 h IV or deep IM in different large muscle masses. Surgical Prophylaxis: 1 g per day IV or deep IM preoperatively.
Cefoperazone Sodium (*)	CEFOBID	Antibacterial	Powd for Inj: 1, 2 g	2 - 4 g daily in equally divided doses q 12 h IM or IV. In severe infections or infections caused by less susceptible organisms, the daily dosage may be increased.
Cefotaxime Sodium (*)	CLAFORAN	Antibacterial	Powd for Inj: 0.5, 1, 2 g Inj (per 50 mL): 1, 2 g	Gonococcal Urethritis & Cervicitis (Males and Females): 500 mg IM as a single dose. Gonorrhea, Rectal: Females: 500 mg IM as a single dose. Males: 1 g IM as a single dose. Uncomplicated Infections: 1 g q 12 h IM or IV. Moderate to Severe Infections: 1 - 2 g q 8 h IM or IV. Infections Commonly Needing Antibiotics in Higher Dosage (e.g., Septicemia): 2 g q 6 - 8 h IV. Life-Threatening Infections: 2 g q 4 h IV.
Cefotetan Disodium (*)	CEFOTAN	Antibacterial	Powd for Inj: 1, 2 g Inj (per 50 mL): 1, 2 g	Urinary Tract Infections: 500 mg q 12 h IM or IV; or 1 - 2 g q 12 - 24 h IM or IV. Skin and Skin Structure Infections: Mild to Moderate: 2 g q 24 h IV or 1 g q 12 h IV or IM

298

Cefoxitin Sodium (*)	MEFOXIN	Antibacterial	Inj (per 50 mL): 1, 2 g Powd for Inj: 1, 2 g	**Severe:** 2 g q 12 h IV. **Other Sites:** 1 - 2 g q 12 h IV or IM. **Severe Infections:** 2 g q 12 h IV. **Life-Threatening Infections:** 3 g q 12 h IV. **Uncomplicated Infections (e.g., Pneumonia, Urinary Tract or Cutaneous Infections:** 1 g q 6 - 8 h IV. **Moderate to Severe Infections:** 1 g q 4 h IV or 2 g q 6 - 8 h IV. **Infections Commonly Needing Higher Dosage (e.g., Gas Gangrene):** 2 g q 4 h IV or 3 g q 6 h IV.
Cefpodoxime Proxetil (*)	VANTIN	Antibacterial	Gran for Susp (per 5 mL): 50, 100 mg Tab: 100, 200 mg	**Pharyngitis & Tonsillitis:** 100 mg q 12 h for 5 - 10 days. **Urinary Tract Infections, Uncomplicated:** 100 mg q 12 h po for 7 days. **Pneumonia:** 200 mg q 12 h po for 14 days. **Bacterial Exacerbation of Chronic Bronchitis:** 200 mg q 12 h po for 10 days. **Skin & Skin Structure Infections:** 400 mg q 12 h po for 7 - 14 days. **Gonococcal Infections:** 200 mg po as a single dose.
Cefprozil (*)	CEFZIL	Antibacterial	Powd for Susp (per 5 mL): 125, 250 mg Tab: 250, 500 mg	**Paryngitis & Tonsillitis:** 500 mg q 24 h po for 10 days. **Acute Sinusitis:** 250 - 500 mg q 12 h po for 10 days. **Lower Respiratory Tract Infections:** 500 mg q 12 h po for 10 days. **Skin & Skin Structure Infections, Uncompl.:** 250 mg q 12 h po for 10 days or 500 mg q 12 - 24 h po for 10 days.
Ceftazidime (*)	FORTAZ, TAZIDIME TAZICEF	Antibacterial	Powd for Inj: 0.5, 1, 2 g Powd for Inj: 1, 2 g	**Usual Dosage:** 1 g q 8 - 12 h IV or IM. **Urinary Tract Infections:** **Uncomplicated:** 250 mg q 12 h IV or IM.

GENERIC NAME	COMMON TRADE NAMES	THERAPEUTIC CATEGORY	PREPARATIONS	COMMON ADULT DOSAGE
Ceftazidime Sodium (*)	FORTAZ	Antibacterial	Inj (per 50 mL): 1, 2 g	**Complicated:** 500 mg q 8 - 12 h IV or IM. **Bone & Joint Infections:** 2 g q 12 h IV. **Pneumonia, Skin & Skin Structure Infections:** 500 mg - 1 g q 8 h IV or IM. **Meningitis, Serious Gynecologic & Intra-Abdominal Infections, and Severe Life-Threatening Infections:** 2 g q 8 h IV.
Ceftibuten (*)	CEDAX	Antibacterial	Cpsl: 400 mg Powd for Susp (per 5 mL): 90, 180 mg	Same dosages as for FORTAZ above. 400 mg once daily po at least 2 h before or 1 h after a meal for 10 days.
Ceftizoxime Sodium (*)	CEFIZOX	Antibacterial	Inj (per 20, 50, or 100 mL): 1, 2 g	**Usual Dosage:** 1 - 2 g q 8 - 12 h IM or IV. **Urinary Tract Infections:** 500 mg q 12 h IM or IV. **Pelvic Inflammatory Disease:** 2 g q 8 h IV. **Other Sites:** 1 g q 8 - 12 h IM or IV. **Severe or Refractory Infections:** 1 g q 8 h IM or IV; or 2 g q 8 - 12 h IM (divided dose in different large muscle masses) or IV. **Life-Threatening Infections:** 3 - 4 g q 8 h IV.
Ceftriaxone Sodium (*)	ROCEPHIN	Antibacterial	Powd for Inj: 250, 500 mg; 1, 2 g	**Usual Dosage:** 1 - 2 g once daily (or in equally divided doses bid) IM or IV. **Gonococcal Infections, Uncomplicated:** 250 mg. IM. One dose. **Meningitis:** 100 mg/kg/day in divided doses q 12 h IM or IV, with or without a loading dose of 75 mg/kg. **Surgical Prophylaxis:** 1 gram IV as a single dose 30 min - 2 h before surgery.
Cefuroxime Axetil (*)	CEFTIN	Antibacterial	Tab: 125, 250, 500 mg Powd for Susp (per 5 mL): 125, 250 mg	**Pharyngitis & Tonsillitis:** 250 mg bid po for 10 days. **Urinary Tract Infections, Uncomplicated:** 125 -

300

Cefuroxime Sodium (*)	KEFUROX, ZINACEF	Antibacterial	Powd for Inj: 0.75, 1.5 g	250 mg bid po for 7 - 10 days. **Acute Bacterial Exacerbations of Chronic Bronchitis and Secondary Bacterial Infections of Acute Bronchitis:** 250 - 500 mg bid po for 10 days. **Usual Dosage:** 750 mg - 1.5 g q 8 h for 5 - 10 days IM or IV. **Bone & Joint Infections:** 1.5 g q 8 h IM or IV. **Life-Threatening Infections or Infections due to Less Susceptible Organisms:** 1.5 g q 6 h IV may be required. **Meningitis:** Up to 3.0 g q 8 h IM or IV. **Gonorrhea:** 1.5 g IM, single dose given at 2 different sites with 1.0 g of probenecid po.
Celecoxib	CELEBREX	Antiinflammatory	Cpsl: 100, 200 mg	**Osteoarthritis:** 200 mg once daily po or 100 mg bid po. **Rheumatoid Arthritis:** 100 - 200 mg bid po.
Cephalexin (*)	KEFLEX	Antibacterial	Powd for Susp (per 5 mL): 125, 250 mg Cpsl: 250, 500 mg	**Usual Dosage:** 250 mg q 6 h po. **Streptococcal Pharyngitis, Skin and Skin Structure Infections and Cystitis:** 500 mg may be used q 12 h po. For cystitis, continue therapy for 7 - 14 days. **Skin or Skin Struct. Infections, Uncomplicated:** 250 - 500 mg bid po for 10 days. **Gonorrhea, Uncomplicated:** 1 g po as a single dose. **Early Lyme Disease:** 500 mg bid po for 20 days.
Cephalexin Hydrochloride (*)	KEFTAB	Antibacterial	Tab: 500 mg	Same dosage as for KEFLEX above.
Cephapirin	CEFADYL	Antibacterial	Powd for Inj: 1 g	**Usual Dosage:** 500 mg - 1 g q 4 - 6 h IV or IM.

GENERIC NAME	COMMON TRADE NAMES	THERAPEUTIC CATEGORY	PREPARATIONS	COMMON ADULT DOSAGE
Sodium (*)				**Serious or Life-Threatening Infections:** Up to 12 g daily IV or IM. Use IV for high doses.
Cephradine (*)	VELOSEF	Antibacterial	**Powd for Susp (per 5 mL):** 125, 250 mg **Cpsl:** 250, 500 mg	**Respiratory Tract, Skin and Skin Structure Infections:** 250 mg q 6 h po or 500 mg q 12 h po. **Lobar Pneumonia:** 500 mg q 6 h po or 1 g q 12 h po. **Urinary Tract Infections:** 500 mg q 12 h po. In more serious urinary tract infections (including prostatitis), 500 mg q 6 h po or 1 g q 12 h po.
Chloramphenicol (*)		Antibacterial	**Cpsl:** 250 mg	50 mg/kg/day in divided doses at 6 h intervals po.
Chloramphenicol Sod. Succinate (*)	CHLOROMYCETIN SODIUM SUCCINATE	Antibacterial	**Powd for Inj:** 100 mg/mL (when reconstituted)	50 mg/kg/day in divided doses at 6 h intervals IV.
Chlorzoxazone	PARAFON FORTE DSC	Skeletal Muscle Relaxant	**Cplt:** 500 mg	500 mg tid or qid po.
Ciprofloxacin (*)	CIPRO I.V.	Antibacterial	**Inj:** 200, 400 mg	**Urinary Tract Infections:** **Mild/Moderate:** 200 mg q 12 h by IV infusion (over 60 minutes) for 7 - 14 days. **Severe/Complicated:** 400 mg q 12 h by IV infusion (over 60 minutes) for 7 - 14 days. **Lower Respiratory Tract, Bone & Joint, and Skin & Skin Structure Infections:** **Mild/Moderate:** 400 mg q 12 h by IV infusion (over 60 minutes) for 7 - 14 days (Bone & Joint = 4 to 6 weeks of therapy). **Severe/Complicated:** 400 mg q 8 h by IV infusion (over 60 minutes) for 7 - 14 days (Bone & Joint = 4 to 6 weeks of therapy). **Acute Sinusitis:** 400 mg q 12 h by IV infusion (over 60 minutes) for 10 days. **Chronic Bacterial Prostatitis:** 400 mg q 12 h by IV infusion (over 60 minutes) for 28 days.

Drug	Brand	Class	Dosage
Ciprofloxacin Hydrochloride (*)	CIPRO	Antibacterial	**Tab:** 100, 250, 500, 750 mg	**Intra-Abdominal Infections:** 400 mg q 12 h by IV infusion (over 60 minutes) for 7 - 14 days. **Inhalational Anthrax (Post-Exposure):** 400 mg q 12 h by IV infusion (over 60 minutes) for 60 days. **Nosocomial Pneumonia:** 400 mg q 8 h by IV infusion (over 60 minutes). **Urinary Tract Infections:** **Acute, Uncomplicated:** 100 mg q 12 h po for 3 days. **Mild/Moderate:** 250 mg q 12 h po for 7 - 14 days. **Severe/Complicated:** 500 mg q 12 h po for 7 - 14 days. **Lower Respiratory Tract and Skin & Skin Structure Infections:** **Mild/Moderate:** 500 mg q 12 h po for 7 - 14 days. **Severe/Complicated:** 750 mg q 12 h for 7 to 14 days. **Bone & Joint Infections:** **Mild/Moderate:** 500 mg q 12 h po for 4 - 6 weeks. **Severe/Complicated:** 750 mg q 12 h po for 4 - 6 weeks. **Infectious Diarrhea:** 500 mg q 12 h po for 5 - 7 days. **Bacterial Prostatitis, Chronic:** 500 mg q 12 h po for 28 days. **Typhoid Fever & Acute Sinusitis:** 500 mg q 12 h po for 10 days. **Gonococcal Infections, Uncomplicated:** 250 mg po (as a single dose).
Clarithromycin (*)	BIAXIN	Antibacterial	**Granules for Susp (per 5 mL):** 125, 250 mg **Tab:** 250, 500 mg	**Usual Dosage:** 250 - 500 mg q 12 h po for 7 - 14 days. *Mycobacterium avium* **Complex (MAC):** 500

GENERIC NAME	COMMON TRADE NAMES	THERAPEUTIC CATEGORY	PREPARATIONS	COMMON ADULT DOSAGE
				mg bid po. **Active Duodenal Ulcer Associated with** *Helicobacter pylori* **Infection:** 500 mg tid po for days 1 - 14 plus omeprazole 40 mg po each AM or ranitidine bismuth citrate 400 mg bid for days 1 - 14.
	BIAXIN XL		Extended-Rel. Tab: 500 mg	**Usual Dosage:** 1000 mg once daily po with food for 7 - 14 days. **Bronchitis:** 1000 mg once daily po with food for 7 days. **Sinusitis:** 1000 mg once daily po with food for 14 days.
Clindamycin Hydrochloride (*)	CLEOCIN HCL	Antibacterial	Cpsl: 75, 150, 300 mg	**Serious Infections:** 150 - 300 mg q 6 h po. **More Severe Infections:** 300 - 450 mg q 6 h po.
Clindamycin Phosphate (*)	CLEOCIN PHOSPHATE	Antibacterial	Inj: 150 mg/mL	**Serious Infections:** 600 - 1200 mg/day IV or IM in 2, 3 or 4 equal doses. **More Severe Infections:** 1200 - 2700 mg/day IV or IM in 2, 3 or 4 equal doses. **Life-Threatening Infections:** Up to 4800 mg/day IV.
Clobetasol Propionate	TEMOVATE	Corticosteroid	Cream, Oint & Gel: 0.05% Scalp Application: 0.05%	Apply topically to affected areas bid. Apply to affected scalp areas bid, AM and PM.
	OLUX		Foam: 0.05%	Apply to affected areas bid, AM and PM.
Clocortolone Pivalate	CLODERM	Corticosteroid	Cream: 0.1%	Apply sparingly to the affected area tid. Rub in gently.
Cloxacillin Sodium (*)		Antibacterial	Cpsl: 250, 500 mg Powd for Solution: 125 mg/5 mL	**Mild to Moderate Infections:** 250 mg q 6 h po. **Severe Infections:** 500 mg q 6 h po.

Codeine Phosphate (*) (C-II)		Opioid Analgesic	Inj (per mL): 30, 60 mg	15 - 60 mg q 4 - 6 h IM, SC or IV.
Codeine Sulfate (C-II)		Opioid Analgesic, Antitussive	Tab: 15, 30, 60 mg	**Analgesia:** 15 - 60 mg q 4 - 6 h po. **Antitussive:** 10 - 20 mg q 4 - 6 h po.
Cyanocobalamin	NASCOBAL	Vitamin	**Metered-Dose Gel:** 500 µg per actuation	500 µg (1 actuation) intranasally once a week.
			Tab: 25, 50, 100, 250 µg	**Deficiency:** 25 - 250 µg daily po.
Cyclobenzaprine Hydrochloride (*)	FLEXERIL	Skeletal Muscle Relaxant	**Tab:** 10 mg	10 mg tid po.
Dalteparin Sodium	FRAGMIN	Anticoagulant	**Solution (per 0.2 mL):** 2,500 (16 mg); 5,000 (32 mg) anti-Xa Units	**Patients Undergoing Abdominal Surgery with Risk of Thromboembolic Complications:** 2,500 Units once daily SC, starting 1 - 2 h prior to surgery and repeated once daily 5 - 10 days postoperatively. In patients with high risk of thromboembolic complications, use 5,000 Units SC in the evening before surgery and repeated once daily for 5 - 10 days postoperatively. **Hip Replacement Surgery:** 2,500 Units SC within 2 h before surgery and 2,500 Units in the evening of the day of surgery (≥ 6 h after the first dose). On the first post-operative day administer 5,000 Units SC once daily for 5 - 10 days. **Unstable Angina/Non-Q-Wave MI:** 120 Units/kg (but not more than 10,000 Units) SC q 12 h with concurrent oral aspirin (75 to 165 mg per day) therapy. Continue until the patient is clinically stabilized (usually 5 - 8 days).
Danaparoid Sodium	ORGARAN	Anticoagulant	**Inj:** 750 anti-Xa Units per 0.6 mL	750 anti-Xa Units bid SC starting 1 - 4 h pre-operatively; then not sooner than 2 h after

GENERIC NAME	COMMON TRADE NAMES	THERAPEUTIC CATEGORY	PREPARATIONS	COMMON ADULT DOSAGE
				surgery. Continue therapy throughout post-operative care until the risk of deep vein thrombosis has diminished (e.g., 7-10 days).
Dantrolene Sodium	DANTRIUM	Skeletal Muscle Relaxant	Cpsl: 25, 50, 100 mg	**Chronic Spasticity:** 25 mg once daily po for 7 days; then 25 mg tid for 7 days; then 50 mg tid for 7 days; then 100 mg tid. Therapy in some patients may require qid dosing. **Malignant Hyperthermia: Preoperatively:** 4 - 8 mg/kg/day po in 3 - 4 divided doses for 1 or 2 days prior to surgery, with the last dose given approx. 3 - 4 h before scheduled surgery. **Post Crisis Follow Up:** 4 - 8 mg/kg/day po in 4 divided doses for 1 - 3 days.
	DANTRIUM INTRAVENOUS		Powd for Inj: 20 mg	**Malignant Hyperthermia: Acute Therapy:** Administer by continuous rapid IV push beginning at a minimum dose of 1 mg/kg, and continuing until the symptoms subside or the max. cumulative dose of 10 mg/kg has been reached. **Preoperatively:** 2.5 mg/kg IV starting approx. 1.25 hours before anticipated anesthesia and infused over 1 h. **Post Crisis Follow Up:** Individualize dose.
Demeclocycline Hydrochloride	DECLOMYCIN	Antibacterial	Tab: 150, 300 mg	150 mg qid po or 300 mg bid po.
Desonide	DESOWEN TRIDESILON	Corticosteroid	Cream, Oint & Lotion: 0.05% Cream & Oint: 0.05%	Apply to the affected areas bid to tid. Apply to the affected areas bid to qid.
Desoximetasone	TOPICORT	Corticosteroid	Cream: 0.05, 0.25% Oint: 0.25% Gel: 0.05%	Apply a thin film to the affected areas bid. Rub in gently.

Dexamethasone	DECADRON	Corticosteroid	Elixir: 0.5 mg/5 mL (5% alcohol) Tab: 0.5, 0.75, 4 mg	Initial dosage varies from 0.75 - 9 mg daily po, depending on the disease being treated. This should be maintained or adjusted until the patient's response is satisfactory.
	MAXIDEX		Ophth Susp: 0.1%	1 - 2 drops in affected eye(s). In severe disease, may use hourly; taper to discontinuation as the inflammation subsides. In mild disease, may use up to 4 - 6 times daily.
Dexamethasone Acetate	DECADRON-LA	Corticosteroid	Inj: 8 mg/mL	Intramuscular Inj: 8 - 16 mg q 1 - 3 weeks. Intralesional Inj: 0.8 - 1.6 mg per inj. site. Intra-articular & Soft Tissue Inj: 4 - 16 mg q 1 - 3 weeks.
Dexamethasone Sodium Phosphate	DECADRON PHOSPHATE	Corticosteroid	Inj: 4 mg/mL	IV and IM Inj: Initial dosage varies from 0.5 - 9 mg daily depending on the disease being treated. This dosage should be maintained or adjusted until the patient's response is satisfactory.
			Inj: 24 mg/mL [for IV use only]	Intra-articular, Intralesional, and Soft Tissue Injection: Varies from 0.2 - 6 mg given from once q 3 - 5 days to once q 2 - 3 weeks.
Diazepam (*) (C-IV)	VALIUM	Antianxiety Agent, Anticonvulsant, Skel. Muscle Relax., Drug for Alcohol Withdrawal	Tab: 2, 5, 10 mg	Anxiety & Adjunct in Convulsive Disorders: 2 - 10 mg bid to qid po. Muscle Spasms: 2 - 10 mg tid to qid po.
			Inj: 5 mg/mL	Anxiety (Moderate): 2 - 5 mg IM or IV. Repeat in 3 - 4 h, if necessary. Anxiety (Severe) and Muscle Spasms: 5 - 10 mg IM or IV. Repeat in 3 - 4 h, if necessary. Preoperative Medication: 10 mg IM (preferred route) before surgery.

307

GENERIC NAME	COMMON TRADE NAMES	THERAPEUTIC CATEGORY	PREPARATIONS	COMMON ADULT DOSAGE
				Status Epilepticus and Severe Recurrent Convulsive Seizures: 5 - 10 mg IV. Repeat at 10 - 15 minute intervals, if necessary, up to a maximum dose of 30 mg. **Acute Alcohol Withdrawal:** Initially 10 mg IM or IV, then 5 - 10 mg in 3 - 4 h, if needed. **Endoscopic Procedures:** Titrate IV dosage to desired sedative response. Generally 10 mg or less is adequate, but up to 20 mg IV may be given.
Diclofenac Potassium (*)	CATAFLAM	Antiinflammatory, Non-Opioid Analgesic	**Tab:** 50 mg	**Osteoarthritis:** 100 - 150 mg/day po in divided doses (50 mg bid or tid). **Rheumatoid Arthritis:** 150 - 200 mg/day po in divided doses (50 mg tid or qid). **Ankylosing Spondylitis:** 100 - 125 mg/day po as: 25 mg qid with an extra 25 mg hs, prn. **Analgesia and Primary Dysmenorrhea:** 50 mg tid or 100 mg initially, followed by 50 mg doses po. Except for the first day when the total dose may be 200 mg, do not exceed 150 mg daily.
Diclofenac Sodium (*)	VOLTAREN	Antiinflammatory	**Delayed-Rel. Tab:** 25, 50, 75 mg	**Osteoarthritis:** 100 - 150 mg/day po in divided doses (50 mg bid or tid or 75 mg bid). **Rheumatoid Arthritis:** 150 - 200 mg/day po in div doses (50 mg tid or qid, or 75 mg bid). **Ankylosing Spondylitis:** 100 - 125 mg/day po as: 25 mg qid with an extra 25 mg hs, prn.
	VOLTAREN-XR	Antiinflammatory	**Extended-Rel. Tab:** 100 mg	**Osteoarthritis & Rheumatoid Arthritis:** 100 mg once daily po.
Dicloxacillin Sodium (*)	DYNAPEN, PATHOCIL	Antibacterial	**Powd for Susp:** 62.5 mg/5 mL **Cpsl:** 250, 500 mg	**Mild to Moderate Infections:** 125 mg q 6 h po. **More Severe Infections:** 250 mg q 6 h po.

Dihydrotachysterol	DHT HYTAKEROL	Vitamin D Analog	**Tab:** 0.125, 0.2, 0.4 mg **Solution:** 0.2 mg/mL **Cpsl:** 0.125 mg	**Initial:** 0.8 - 2.4 mg po daily for several days. **Maintenance:** 0.2 - 1.75 mg daily po. The average dose is 0.6 mg daily po.
Dipyridamole	PERSANTINE	Platelet Aggregation	**Tab:** 25, 50, 75 mg	75 - 100 mg qid po.
Dirithromycin	DYNABAC	Antibacterial	**Enteric-Coated Tab:** 250 mg	500 mg once daily po with for 7 - 14 days. Administer with food or within 1 h of eating.
Docusate Calcium	SURFAK LIQUIGELS	Stool Softener	**Cpsl:** 240 mg	240 mg daily po.
Docusate Sodium	COLACE	Stool Softener	**Syrup:** 20 mg/5 mL **Cpsl:** 50, 100 mg	50 - 200 mg daily po.
	EX-LAX STOOL SOFTENER		**Cplt:** 100 mg	100 mg once daily to tid po.
	PHILLIPS LIQUI-GELS		**Liqui-Gel:** 100 mg	100 mg once daily to tid po.
Doxycycline Calcium (*)	VIBRAMYCIN	Antibacterial, Antimalarial	**Syrup:** 50 mg/5 mL	**Usual Dosage:** 100 mg q 12 h po for the first day, followed by a maintenance dose of 100 mg/day given as 50 mg q 12 h or 100 mg once daily. **Urinary Tract Infections:** 100 mg q 12 h po. **Malaria Prophylaxis:** 100 mg once daily po.

GENERIC NAME	COMMON TRADE NAMES	THERAPEUTIC CATEGORY	PREPARATIONS	COMMON ADULT DOSAGE
Doxycycline Hydate (*)	VIBRAMYCIN VIBRA-TAB	Antibacterial, Antimalarial	**Cpsl:** 50, 100 mg **Tab:** 100 mg	Same dosages as for VIBRAMYCIN Syrup.
	DORYX		**Cpsl (with coated pellets):** 100 mg	Same dosages as for VIBRAMYCIN Syrup.
	VIBRAMYCIN INTRAVENOUS	Antibacterial	**Powd for Inj:** 100, 200 mg	**Usual Dosage:** 200 mg on the first day given in 1 or 2 IV infusions, then 100 - 200 mg a day, with 200 mg given in 1 or 2 infusions. **Syphilis:** 300 mg daily by IV infusion for at least 10 days.
	PERIOSTAT	Periodontitis Drug	**Tab:** 20 mg	20 mg bid po, 1 h before or 2 h after meals.
Doxycycline Monohydrate (*)	VIBRAMYCIN	Antibacterial, Antimalarial	**Powd for Susp:** 25 mg/5 mL	Same dosages as for VIBRAMYCIN Syrup.
Enoxacin (*)	PENETREX	Antibacterial	**Tab:** 200, 400 mg	**Urinary Tract Infections (Uncomplicated):** 200 mg q 12 h po for 7 days. **Urinary Tract Infections (Complicated):** 400 mg q 12 h po for 14 days. **Gonorrhea (Uncomplicated):** 400 mg po as a single dose.
Erythromycin (*)	ERY-TAB ERYC	Antibacterial	**Delayed-Rel. Tab:** 250, 333, 500 mg **Delayed-Rel. Cpsl:** 250 mg	**Usual Dosage:** 250 mg qid po; 333 mg q 8 h po; or 500 mg bid (q 12 h) po. **Streptococcal Infections:** Administer the usual dosage for at least 10 days.
	ERYTHROMYCIN BASE FILMTAB		**Tab:** 250, 500 mg	**Primary Syphilis:** 20 - 40 g po in divided doses over a period of 10 - 15 days.
	PCE		**Dispersable Tab:** 333, 500 mg	**Acute Pelvic Inflammatory Disease due to N. gonorrhoeae:** After initial treatment with erythromycin lactobionate, give 250 mg q 6 h po for 7 days or 333 mg q 8 h for 7 days. **Urogenital Infections during pregnancy and**

Drug		Category	Forms	Indications / Dosage
Erythromycin Estolate (*)	ILOSONE	Antibacterial	Susp (per 5 mL): 125, 250 mg Cpsl: 250 mg Tab: 500 mg	**Uncomplicated Urethral, Endocervical, or Rectal Infections due to C. trachomatis:** 500 mg qid po or 666 mg q 8 h po for at least 7 days. **Dysenteric Amebiasis:** 250 mg qid po or 333 mg q 8 h po for 10 - 14 days. **Legionnaires Disease:** 1 - 4 g daily po in divided doses.
Erythromycin Ethylsuccinate (*)	E.E.S.	Antibacterial	Gran for Susp (per 5 mL): 200 mg Susp (per 5 mL): 200, 400 mg Tab: 400 mg	**Usual Dosage:** 250 mg q 6 h po or 500 mg q 12 h po. **Streptococcal Infections:** Administer the usual dosage for at least 10 days. **Primary Syphilis:** 20 - 40 g po in divided doses over a period of 10 - 15 days. **Urogenital Infections during pregnancy and Uncomplicated Urethral, Endocervical, or Rectal Infections due to C. trachomatis:** 500 mg qid po for at least 7 days. **Dysenteric Amebiasis:** 250 mg qid po for 10 to 14 days. **Legionnaires Disease:** 1 - 4 g daily po in divided doses.
	ERYPED		Powd for Susp (per 5 mL): 200, 400 mg Chewable Tab: 200 mg	**Usual Dosage:** 400 mg q 6 h po or 800 mg q 12 h po. **Streptococcal Infections:** Administer the usual dosage for at least 10 days. **Primary Syphilis:** 48 - 64 g po in divided doses over a period of 10 - 15 days. **Urethritis due to C. trachomatis or U. urealyticum:** 800 mg tid po for 7 days. **Intestinal Amebiasis:** 400 mg qid po for 10 to 14 days. **Legionnaires Disease:** 1.6 - 4 g daily po in divided doses.
Erythromycin Gluceptate (*)	ILOTYCIN GLUCEPTATE	Antibacterial	Powd for Inj: 1 g	**Usual Dosage:** 5 - 20 mg/kg/day by continuous IV infusion or in divided doses q 6 h IV. **Acute Pelvic Inflammatory Disease due to N.**

GENERIC NAME	COMMON TRADE NAMES	THERAPEUTIC CATEGORY	PREPARATIONS	COMMON ADULT DOSAGE
Erythromycin Lactobionate (*)	ERYTHROCIN IV	Antibacterial	Powd for Inj: 500 mg; 1 g	*gonorrhoeae:* 500 mg q 6 h IV for at least 3 days, followed by 250 mg of oral erythromycin q 6 h for 7 days. **Severe Infections:** 15-20 mg/kg/day by contin. IV infusion or by intermittent IV infusion in 20 - 60 min periods at intervals of ≤ 6 h.
Erythromycin Stearate (*)	ERYTHROCIN STEARATE	Antibacterial	Tab: 250, 500 mg	**Usual Dosage:** 250 mg q 6 h po or 500 mg q 12 h po on an empty stomach or ac. **Streptococcal Infections:** Administer the usual dosage for at least 10 days. **Acute Pelvic Inflammatory Disease due to** *N. gonorrhoeae:* After initial treatment with erythromycin lactobionate, give 250 mg q 6 h po for 7 days. **Urogenital Infections during pregnancy and Uncomplicated Urethral, Endocervical, or Rectal Infections due to C. trachomatis:** 500 mg qid po for at least 7 days. **Intestinal Amebiasis:** 250 mg qid po for 10 to 14 days.
Etidronate Disodium	DIDRONEL	Bone Stabilizer	Tab: 200, 400 mg	**Paget's Disease:** Initially, 5 mg/kg daily po, not to exceed 6 months. May increase to 10 mg/kg daily po, not to exceed 6 months or to 11 - 20 mg/kg daily po, not to exceed 3 months. Take on an empty stomach 2 h ac.
	DIDRONEL I.V. INFUSION		Inj: 300 mg/6 mL	7.5 mg/kg daily by IV infusion (over at least 2 h) for 3 days. Daily dose must be diluted in at least 250 mL of sterile normal saline.
Etodolac	LODINE	Non-Opioid Analgesic, Antiinflammatory	Cpsl: 200, 300 mg Tab: 400, 500 mg	**Analgesia:** 200 - 400 mg q 6 - 8 h po. **Osteoarthritis & Rheumatoid Arthritis:** Initially, 300 mg bid or tid po, 400 mg bid po, or 500 mg bid po. Adjust dosage within 600 to 1200 mg/day po prn for maintenance.

	LODINE XL	Antiinflammatory	Extended-Rel. Tab: 400, 500, 600 mg	Osteoarthritis & Rheumatoid Arthritis: 400 to 1000 mg once daily po.
Fenoprofen Calcium (*)	NALFON	Non-Opioid Analgesic, Antiinflammatory	Cpsl: 200, 300 mg; Tab: 600 mg	Analgesia: 200 mg q 4 - 6 h po, prn. Rheumatoid Arthritis and Osteoarthritis: 300 to 600 mg tid to qid po.
Fentanyl (*) (C-II)	DURAGESIC	Opioid Analgesic	Transdermal: rate = 25, 50, 75, 100 µg/hr	Individualize dosage. Each system may be worn for up to 72 h.
Fentanyl Citrate (*) (C-II)	SUBLIMAZE	Opioid Analgesic	Inj: 50 µg/mL (as the base)	2 - 50 µg/kg IM or IV.
	FENTANYL ORALET	Opioid Analgesic	Lozenge: 100, 200, 300, 400 µg	Administer only in a hospital setting. Individualize dosage. Fentanyl transmucosal doses of 5 µg/kg (400 µg) provide effects similar to usual doses of fentanyl citrate given IM, i.e., 0.75 - 1.25 µg/kg. Oral administration should begin 20 - 40 minutes prior to anticipated need of desired effect.
	ACTIQ		Lozenge on a Stick: 200, 400, 600, 800, 1200, 1600 µg	Initial dose to treat episodes of breakthrough cancer pain should be 200 µg consumed over a 15-min. period. Prescribe an initial titration supply of six 200 µg units. Advise patients to use all units before increasing to a higher dose. Redosing should not occur more often than q 30 min. Dose increases may be occur after evaluation over several episodes of breakthrough cancer pain.
Flunisolide	AEROBID	Corticosteroid	Aerosol: 250 µg/spray	2 inhalations bid AM and PM.
	NASALIDE, NASAREL		Spray: 25 µg/spray	2 sprays in each nostril bid.
Fluocinolone Acetonide	SYNALAR	Corticosteroid	Cream: 0.01, 0.025% Oint: 0.025% Solution: 0.01%	Apply as a thin film bid - qid.

313

GENERIC NAME	COMMON TRADE NAMES	THERAPEUTIC CATEGORY	PREPARATIONS	COMMON ADULT DOSAGE
	SYNALAR-HP		Cream: 0.2%	Apply as a thin film bid - qid.
Fluorometholone	FML	Corticosteroid	Ophth Susp: 0.1%	1 drop into affected eye(s) bid - qid. During the initial 24 - 48 hours, the frequency of dosing may be increased if necessary.
	FML FORTE		Ophth Susp: 0.25%	1 drop into affected eye(s) bid - qid.
	FML		Ophth Oint: 0.1%	Apply 1/2 inch ribbon to eye(s) q 4 h for the 1st 24 - 48 h. When a favorable response is observed, reduce dosage to 1 - 3 times daily.
Fluorometholone Acetate	FLAREX	Corticosteroid	Ophth Susp: 0.1%	1 - 2 drops into affected eye(s) qid. May initiate with 2 drops q 2 h during the initial 24 - 48 hours; then, the frequency of dosing may be decreased.
Flurandrenolide	CORDRAN	Corticosteroid	Cream & Oint: 0.025, 0.05% Lotion: 0.05% Tape: 4 mcg/cm²	Apply as a thin film to affected areas bid - tid and rub in gently. Apply to affected areas; replace q 12 h.
Flurbiprofen (*)	ANSAID	Antiinflammatory	Tab: 50, 100 mg	200 - 300 mg daily, given bid, tid or qid po.
Flurbiprofen Sodium	OCUFEN	Antiinflammatory (Topical)	Ophth Solution: 0.03%	1 drop in eye q 30 minutes, beginning 2 h before surgery (total of 4 drops).
Fluticasone Propionate	CUTIVATE	Corticosteroid	Oint: 0.005% Cream: 0.05%	Apply a thin film to affected skin areas bid. Rub in gently.
	FLONASE	Corticosteroid	Nasal Spray: 50 µg/spray	Initially, 2 sprays in each nostril once daily or 1 spray in each nostril twice daily (morning and evening). May decrease to 1 spray in each nostril once daily based on response. For Adolescents over 12 yrs: Initially, 1 spray in each nostril once daily; may increase to 2 sprays in each nostril once daily, then may decrease to 1 spray in each nostril once daily based on response.

Folic Acid		Vitamin	**Usual Therapeutic Dose**: up to 1 mg daily po.
Furazolidone	FUROXONE	Antibacterial	100 mg qid po.
Gatifloxacin Sesquihydrate	TEQUIN	Antibacterial	**Urinary Tract Infections (Complicated), Bronchitis, Pyelonephritis**: 400 mg once daily po or by slow IV infusion for 7 - 10 days. **Urinary Tract Infections (Uncomplicated)**: 200 or 400 mg po or by slow IV infusion as a single dose for 3 days. **Community-Acquired Pneumonia**: 400 mg once daily po or by slow IV infusion for 7 - 14 days. **Acute Sinusitis**: 400 mg once daily po or by slow IV infusion for 10 days. **Gonorrhea**: 400 mg po or by slow IV infusion as a single dose.
Halcinonide	HALOG	Corticosteroid	Apply to affected areas bid to tid.
Halobetasol Propionate	ULTRAVATE	Corticosteroid	Apply a thin layer to affected skin once or twice daily. Rub in gently and completely.
Heparin Sodium (*)		Anticoagulant	**Deep SC**: 5000 units IV, followed by 10,000 to 20,000 units SC. Then 8,000 - 10,000 units q 8 h or 15,000 - 20,000 units q 12 h. **Intermittent IV**: 10,000 units undiluted or in 50 - 100 mL of 0.9% sodium chloride injection. Then 5,000 - 10,000 units undiluted or in sodium chloride injection q 4 - 6 h. **IV Infusion**: 5,000 units IV; then 20,000 to 40,000 units/24 h in 1,000 mL of 0.9% NaCl injection by continuous IV infusion.

Tab: 0.4, 0.8, 1 mg

Liquid: 50 mg/15 mL
Tab: 100 mg

Tab: 200, 400 mg
Inj: 10 mg/mL

Cream, Oint & Solution: 0.1%

Cream & Oint: 0.05%

Inj: 1,000 - 40,000 units/mL

GENERIC NAME	COMMON TRADE NAMES	THERAPEUTIC CATEGORY	PREPARATIONS	COMMON ADULT DOSAGE
Hyaluronate Sodium	HYALGAN	Treatment of pain in osteoarthritis	Solution: 20 mg/2.0mL syringe	Intra-articular injection. Five injections given at weekly intervals as a treatment cycle.
Hydrocortisone Acetate	HYDROCORTONE ACETATE	Corticosteroid	Inj (per mL): 25, 50 mg [low solubility; provides a prolonged effect]	**Only for Intra-articular, Intralesional and Soft Tissue Injection:** Dose and frequency of injection are variable and must be individualized on the basis of the disease and the response of the patient. The initial dosage varies from 5 - 75 mg a day.
Hydrocortisone Sodium Phosphate	HYDROCORTONE PHOSPHATE	Corticosteroid	Inj: 50 mg/mL [water soluble; rapid onset; short duration]	**For IV, IM & SC Injection:** Dose requirements vary and must be individualized on the basis of the disease and the response of the patient. Initial daily dose: from 15 - 240 mg.
Hydrocortisone Sodium Succinate	SOLU-CORTEF	Corticosteroid	Powd for Inj: 100, 250, 500, 1000 mg	100 - 500 mg IM, IV, or by IV infusion. Repeat at intervals of 2, 4, or 6 h.
Hydrocortisone Valerate	WESTCORT	Corticosteroid	Cream & Oint: 0.2%	Apply to affected areas as a thin film bid to tid.
Hydromorphone Hydrochloride (*) (C-II)	DILAUDID	Opioid Analgesic	Tab: 2, 3, 4, 8 mg Oral Liquid: 5 mg/5 mL Inj: 1, 2, 4 mg/mL Rectal Suppos: 3 mg	2 mg q 4 - 6 h po, prn. More severe pain may require 4 mg or more q 4 - 6 h po. 2.5 - 10 mg (2.5 - 10 mL) q 3 - 6 h po. 1 - 2 mg q 4 - 6 h SC or IM, prn. For IV use, give dose slowly over at least 2 - 3 minutes. Insert 1 suppository rectally q 6 - 8 h.
Hydromorphone Hydrochloride	DILAUDID-HP	Opioid Analgesic	Inj: 10 mg/mL Powd for Inj: 250 mg	1 - 2 mg q 4 - 6 h SC or IM.

Hylan G-F20	SYNVISC	Treatment of pain in osteoarthritis	16 mg/2 mL syringe (Hylan Polymers)	2 mL intra-articular injections once a week (one week apart) for a total of three injections.
Ibuprofen (*)	ADVIL, MOTRIN IB, NUPRIN	Non-Opioid Analgesic; Antipyretic	**Tab**: 200 mg	200 - 400 mg q 4 - 6 h po.
	MOTRIN MIGRAINE PAIN	Non-Opioid Analgesic	**Cplt**: 200 mg	200 - 400 mg q 4 - 6 h po.
	MOTRIN	Non-Opioid Analgesic; Antiinflammatory	**Susp**: 100 mg/5 mL **Tab**: 400, 600, 800 mg	**Analgesia**: 400 mg q 4 - 6 h prn pain. **Dysmenorrhea**: 400 mg q 4 h po prn pain. **Rheumatoid Arthritis and Osteoarthritis**: 1200 to 3200 mg daily po in divided doses (300 mg qid or 400, 600, or 800 mg tid or qid).
Indomethacin (*)	INDOCIN	Antiinflammatory	**Susp**: 25 mg/5 mL **Cpsl**: 25, 50 mg **Rectal Suppos**: 50 mg	**Rheumatoid Arthritis**: 25 mg bid or tid po pc; if well tolerated, increase the daily dosage by 25 or 50 mg. In persistent night pain or AM stiffness, giving a large portion of the daily dose (up to 100 mg) hs po or by suppository may be helpful. **Acute Painful Shoulder**: 75 - 150 mg daily po pc in 3 - 4 divided doses for 7 - 14 days. **Acute Gout**: 50 mg tid po pc until pain is tolerable.
	INDOCIN SR		**Sustained-Rel. Cpsl**: 75 mg	75 mg daily po.
Ketoconazole (*)	NIZORAL	Antifungal	**Tab**: 200 mg	200 mg once daily po. In very severe infections, 400 mg once daily po.
			Cream: 2% **Shampoo**: 2%	Apply topically once daily. Shampoo twice a week for 4 weeks with at least 3 days between shampooing; then shampoo intermittently prn.

GENERIC NAME	COMMON TRADE NAMES	THERAPEUTIC CATEGORY	PREPARATIONS	COMMON ADULT DOSAGE
	NIZORAL A-D	Antidandruff Shampoo	**Shampoo:** 1%	Shampoo twice a week for up to 8 weeks with at least 3 days between shampooing; then shampoo intermittently prn.
Ketoprofen (*)	ORUDIS KT ORUDIS	Non-Opioid Analgesic, Antiinflammatory	**Tab:** 12.5 mg **Cpsl:** 25, 50, 75 mg	12.5 - 25 mg q 4 - 6 h po prn. **Analgesia & Dysmenorrhea:** 25 - 50 mg q 6 - 8 h po. **Rheumatoid Arthritis & Osteoarthritis:** 75 mg tid po or 50 mg qid po.
Ketoprofen (*)	ORUVAIL	Antiinflammatory	**Extended-Rel. Cpsl:** 100, 150, 200 mg	**Rheumatoid Arthritis & Osteoarthritis:** 200 mg once daily po.
Ketorolac Tromethamine (*)	ACULAR	Antiinflammatory (Topical)	**Ophth Solution:** 0.5%	1 drop into affected eye(s) qid.
	TORADOL IV/IM	Non-Opioid Analgesic	**Inj (per mL):** 15, 30 mg	**Single-Dose Treatment (IM or IV):** **< 65 yrs:** 1 dose of 60 mg IM or 30 mg IV. **≥ 65 yrs, renally impaired, or under 50 kg (110 lbs):** 1 dose of 30 mg IM or 15 mg IV. **Multiple-Dose Treatment (IM or IV):** **< 65 yrs:** 30 mg q 6 h IM or IV, not to exceed 120 mg per day. **≥ 65 yrs, renally impaired, or under 50 kg (110 lbs):** 15 mg q 6 h IM or IV, not to exceed 60 mg per day. · The IV bolus dose must be given over no less than 15 seconds.
	TORADOL ORAL		**Tab:** 10 mg	Indicated only as continuation therapy to TORADOL IV/IM. The maximum combined duration of use (parenteral and oral) is 5 days. **< 65 yrs:** 20 mg po as a first dose for those who received 60 mg IM (single dose), 30 mg IV (single dose), or 30 mg (multiple

318

			dose) of TORADOL.[M/M], followed by 10 mg q 4 - 6 h po, not to exceed 40 mg/day. **≥ 65 yrs, renally impaired, or under 50 kg (110 lbs):** 10 mg po as a first dose for those who received 30 mg IM or 15 mg IV (single dose), or 15 mg (multiple dose) of TORADOL [M/M], followed by 10 mg q 4 - 6 h po, not to exceed 40 mg/day.
Levofloxacin (*)	QUIXIN	Antibacterial	**Ophth Solution:** 0.5%	Instill 1 - 2 drops in the affected eye(s) q 2 h while awake, up to 8 times a day on days 1 and 2. Instill 1 - 2 drops in the affected eye(s) q 4 h while, up to 4 times daily on days 3 - 7.
Levofloxacin (*)	LEVAQUIN	Antibacterial	**Tab:** 250, 500, 750 mg **Inj:** 25 mg/mL	**Bronchitis:** 500 mg once daily po or by IV infusion (over 60 min) for 7 days. **Pneumonia:** 500 mg once daily po or by IV infusion (over 60 min) for 7 - 14 days. **Sinusitis:** 500 mg once daily po or by IV infusion (over 60 min) for 10 - 14 days. **Skin & Skin Structure Infections (Uncomplicated):** 500 mg once daily po or by IV infusion (over 60 min) for 7 - 10 days. **Skin & Skin Structure Infections (Complicated):** 750 mg once daily po or by IV infusion (over 90 min) for 7 - 10 days. **Urinary Tract Infections (Complicated) and Pyelonephritis:** 250 mg once daily po or by IV infusion (over 60 min) for 10 days. **Urinary Tract Infections (Uncomplicated):** 250 mg once daily po for 3 days.
Levorphanol Tartrate (*) (C-II)	LEVO-DROMORAN	Opioid Analgesic	**Tab:** 2 mg **Inj:** 2 mg/mL	2 mg po q 6 - 8 h prn. May be increased to 3 mg q 6 - 8 h if needed. 1 - 2 mg IM or SC q 6 - 8 pm.
Linezolid	ZYVOX	Antibacterial	**Inj:** 2 mg/mL **Tab:** 400, 600 mg **Powd for Solution:** 100 mg/5 mL	**Vancomycin-resistant *Enterococcus faecium* Infections:** 600 mg IV (over 30 - 120 min) or po q 12 h for 14 - 28 days.

319

GENERIC NAME	COMMON TRADE NAMES	THERAPEUTIC CATEGORY	PREPARATIONS	COMMON ADULT DOSAGE
				Nosocomial Pneumonia, Complicated Skin and Skin Structure Infections, and Community-acquired Pneumonia: 600 mg IV (over 30 to 120 min) or po q 12 h for 10 - 14 days. Uncomplicated Skin and Skin Structure Infections: 400 mg IV (over 30 - 120 min) or po q 12 h for 10 - 10 days.
Lomefloxacin Hydrochloride (*)	MAXAQUIN	Antibacterial	Tab: 400 mg	Lower Respiratory Tract and Urinary Tract Infections (Uncomplicated): 400 mg once daily po for 10 days. Urinary Tract Infections, Complicated: 400 mg once daily po for 14 days.
Loracarbef (*)	LORABID	Antibacterial	Powd for Susp (per 5 mL): 100, 200 mg Cpsl: 200, 400 mg	Lower Resp. Tract Infect. (Except Pneumonia): 200 - 400 mg q 12 h po for 7 days. Pneumonia: 400 mg q 12 h po for 14 days. Upper Respiratory Tract Infections: 200 - 400 mg q 12 h po for 10 days. Skin and Skin Structure Infections: 200 mg q 12 h po for 7 days. Urinary Tract Infections (Uncomplicated Cystitis): 200 mg q 24 h po for 7 days. Urinary Tract Infections (Uncomplicated Pyelonephritis): 400 mg q 12 h po for 14 days.
Mafenide Acetate	SULFAMYLON	Burn Preparation	Cream: 85 mg/g	Apply to the clean and debrided wound with a sterile gloved hand, once or twice daily, to a thickness of about 1/16 in.
Meclofenamate Sodium		Non-Opioid Analgesic, Antiinflammatory	Cpsl: 50, 100 mg	Analgesia: 50 - 100 mg q 4 - 6 h po. Dysmenorrhea: 100 mg tid po, for up to 6 days, starting at the onset of menses. Rheumatoid Arthritis & Osteoarthritis: 200 to 400 mg daily po in 3 or 4 equal doses.

320

Generic	Brand	Class	Strengths	Dosage
Mefenamic Acid (*)	PONSTEL	Non-Opioid Analgesic	**Cpsl:** 250 mg	500 mg po, then 250 mg q 6 h po with food.
Meloxicam	MOBIC	Antiinflammatory	**Tab:** 7.5, 15 mg	7.5 mg once daily po.
Meperidine Hydrochloride (*) (C-II)	DEMEROL	Opioid Analgesic	**Tab:** 50, 100 mg **Syrup:** 50 mg/5 mL **Inj (per mL):** 25, 50, 75, 100 mg	**Analgesia:** 50 - 150 mg q 3 - 4 h po, IM or SC. **Preoperatively:** 50 - 100 mg IM or SC, 30 - 90 minutes prior to anesthesia. **Obstetrical Analgesia:** 50 - 100 mg IM or SC when pain becomes regular; may repeat at 1 - 3 hour intervals.
Meropenem (*)	MERREM IV	Antibacterial	**Powd for Inj:** 0.5, 1 g	1 g q 8 h by IV infusion (over 15 - 30 min) or as an IV bolus (5 - 20 mL) over 3 - 5 min.
Methadone Hydrochloride (*) (C-II)	DOLOPHINE HYDROCHLORIDE	Opioid Analgesic	**Tab:** 5, 10 mg **Inj:** 10 mg/mL	2.5 - 10 mg q 3 - 4 h po, IM or SC prn pain.
Methocarbamol (*)	ROBAXIN	Skeletal Muscle Relaxant	**Tab:** 500 mg	**Initial:** 1500 mg qid po. **Maintenance:** 1000 mg qid po.
	ROBAXIN-750		**Tab:** 750 mg	**Initial:** 1500 mg qid po. **Maintenance:** 750 mg q 4 h po or 1500 mg tid po.
Methylprednisolone	MEDROL	Corticosteroid	**Tab:** 2, 4, 8, 16, 24, 32 mg	Initial dosage varies from 4 - 48 mg daily po, depending on the disease being treated. This dosage should be maintained or adjusted until the patient's response is satisfactory.
Methylprednisolone Acetate	DEPO-MEDROL	Corticosteroid	**Inj (per mL):** 40, 80 mg	Initial dosage varies from 20 - 80 mg weekly to monthly, depending on the disease being treated; the dosage may be given intra-articularly or IM. The dosage should be maintained or adjusted until the patient's response is satisfactory.

GENERIC NAME	COMMON TRADE NAMES	THERAPEUTIC CATEGORY	PREPARATIONS	COMMON ADULT DOSAGE
Methylprednisolone Sodium Succinate	SOLU-MEDROL	Corticosteroid	**Powd for Inj:** 40, 125, 500 mg; 1, 2 g	30 mg/kg IV (administered over at least 30 minutes) q 4 - 6 h for 48 hours.
Mezlocillin Sodium (*)	MEZLIN	Antibacterial	**Powd for Inj:** 1, 2, 3, 4 g	**Urinary Tract Infections (Uncomplicated):** 100 to 125 mg/kg as 1.5 - 2.0 g q 6 h IV or IM. **Urinary Tract Infections (Complicated):** 150 to 200 mg/kg as 3.0 g q 6 h IV. **Intra-Abdominal, Gynecological, Skin & Skin Structure Infections, Lower Respiratory Infections and Septicemia:** 225 - 300 mg/kg as 3.0 g q 4 h IV or 4.0 g q 6 h IV. **Life-Threatening Infections:** Up to 350 mg/kg/day as 4.0 g q 4 h. **Gonococcal Infections (Acute, Uncomplicated):** 1 - 2 g IV or IM + 1 g of probenecid at the time of dosing or up to 30 minutes before.
Morphine Sulfate (*) (C-II)	ASTRAMORPH/PF, DURAMORPH	Opioid Analgesic	**Inj (per mL):** 0.5, 1 mg	IV: 2 - 10 mg/70 kg. **Epidural:** Initially, 5 mg in the lumbar region; after 1 hour, incremental doses of 1 - 2 mg at interval sufficient to assess effectiveness may be given carefully. Max: 10 mg/24 h. **Intrathecal:** 0.2 - 1 mg in the lumbar area.
	INFUMORPH		**Inj (per mL):** 10, 25 mg	**Intrathecal Infusion:** Initially, 0.2 - 1 mg/day (patients with no opioid tolerance) and 1 - 10 mg/day (opioid tolerance) in the lumbar area. **Epidural Infusion:** 3.5 - 7.5 mg/day (patients with no opioid tolerance) and 4.5 - 10 mg/day (opioid tolerance).
	KADIAN		**Sustained-Rel. Cpsl:** 20, 50, 100 mg	Variable po dosages based on patient tolerance to opioids and type of conversion, e.g., from oral morphine, parenteral morphine, or other opioid analgesics. Commonly used q 24 h.
	MS CONTIN		**Controlled-Rel. Tab:** 15, 30,	Variable po dosages based on patient tolerance

ORAMORPH SR	60, 100, 200 mg **Sustained-Rel. Tab:** 15, 30, 60, 100 mg	to opioids and type of conversion, e.g., from oral morphine, parenteral morphine, or other opioid analgesics. Commonly used q 12 h.
MSIR	**Solution (per 5 mL):** 10, 20 mg **Conc Solution:** 20 mg/mL **Cpsl & Tab:** 15, 30 mg	5 - 30 mg q 4 h po prn pain.
RMS	**Rectal Suppos:** 5, 10, 20, 30 mg	10 - 20 mg q 4 h rectally.
ROXANOL	**Oral Solution:** 20 mg/mL	10 - 30 mg q 4 h po prn pain.
ROXANOL 100	**Oral Solution:** 100 mg/5 mL	10 - 30 mg q 4 h po prn pain.

GENERIC NAME	COMMON TRADE NAMES	THERAPEUTIC CATEGORY	PREPARATIONS	COMMON ADULT DOSAGE
Moxifloxacin Hydrochloride	AVELOX	Antibacterial	Tab: 400 mg	**Acute Bacterial Exacerbation of Chronic Bronchitis:** 400 mg once daily po for 5 days. **Community-Acquired Pneumonia and Acute Bacterial Sinusitis:** 400 mg once daily po for 10 days. **Skin & Skin Structure Infections (Uncomplic.):** 400 mg once daily po for 7 days.
Nabumetone (*)	RELAFEN	Antiinflammatory	Tab: 500, 750 mg	Initially 1000 mg po as a single dose with or without food. Dosage may be increased to 1500 - 2000 mg/day as a single dose or in 2 divided doses.
Nafcillin Sodium (*)		Antibacterial	Cpsl: 250 mg	**Mild to Moderate Infections:** 250 - 500 mg q 4 to 6 h po. **Severe Infections:** 1000 mg q 4 - 6 h po.
Nalbuphine Hydrochloride (*)	NUBAIN	Opioid Analgesic	Inj (per mL): 10, 20 mg	10 mg/70 kg SC, IM, or IV; dose may be repeated q 3 - 6 h prn.
Nalmefene Hydrochloride	REVEX	Opioid Antagonist	Inj (per mL): 100 µg, 1.0 mg	**Opioid Overdose (Known or Suspected):** Use the 1.0 mg/mL strength. **Non-Opioid Dependent Patients:** 0.5 mg/70

GENERIC NAME	COMMON TRADE NAMES	THERAPEUTIC CATEGORY	PREPARATIONS	COMMON ADULT DOSAGE
				kg IM, SC, or IV. If needed, this may be followed by a 2nd dose of 1.0 mg/70 kg, 2 - 5 minutes later. **Suspected Opioid-Dependent Patients:** An initial challenge dose of 0.1 mg/70 kg should be used. If no evidence of withdrawal occurs, use the above dosage. **Postoperative Opioid Respiratory Depression:** Use the **100 μg/mL** strength. Initially 0.25 μg/kg IM, SC or IV, followed by 0.25 μg/kg incremental doses at 2 - 5 minute intervals, stopping as soon as the desired degree of opioid reversal occurs.
Naloxone Hydrochloride (*)	NARCAN	Opioid Antagonist	Inj (per mL): 0.4, 1 mg	**Opioid Overdose (Known or Suspected):** Initially, 0.4 - 2 mg IV. Dose may be repeated at 2 - 3 min intervals. Max: 10 mg. **Postoperative Opioid Respiratory Depression:** 0.1 - 0.2 mg IV at 2 - 3 minute intervals. Doses may be repeated in 1 - 2 hours.
Naltrexone Hydrochloride (*)	REVIA	Opioid Antagonist	Tab: 50 mg	50 mg once daily for most patients.
Naproxen (*)	NAPROSYN	Non-Opioid Analgesic, Antiinflammatory	Susp: 125 mg/5 mL. Tab: 250, 375, 500 mg	**Analgesia, Dysmenorrhea, Acute Tendonitis and Bursitis:** 500 mg po, followed by 250 mg po q 6 - 8 h prn. **Acute Gout:** 750 mg po, followed by 250 mg po q 8 h until the attack has subsided. **Rheumatoid Arthritis, Osteoarthritis and Ankylosing Spondylitis:** 250 - 500 mg bid po, morning and evening. **Juvenile Arthritis:** 5 mg/kg bid po.
	EC-NAPROSYN	Antiinflammatory	Delayed-Rel. Tab: 375, 500 mg	**Rheumatoid Arthritis, Osteoarthritis and Ankylosing Spondylitis:** 375 - 500 mg bid po, morning and evening.

Naproxen Sodium	ALEVE	Non-Opioid Analgesic, Antipyretic	Cplt, Tab & Gelcap: 220 mg	**Analgesia & Fever:** 220 mg q 8 - 12 h po with a full glass of liquid, while symptoms persist or 440 mg initially, followed by 220 mg 12 h later.
	ANAPROX ANAPROX DS	Non-Opioid Analgesic, Antiinflammatory	Tab: 275 mg Tab: 550 mg	**Analgesia, Dysmenorrhea, Acute Tendonitis and Bursitis:** 550 mg po, followed by 275 mg po q 6 - 8 h pm. **Acute Gout:** 825 mg po, followed by 275 mg po q 8 h until the attack has subsided. **Rheumatoid Arthritis, Osteoarthritis and Ankylosing Spondylitis:** 275 or 550 mg bid po, morning and evening.
	NAPRELAN	Non-Opioid Analgesic, Antiinflammatory	Controlled-Rel. Tab: 412.5 550 mg (equivalent to 375 and 500 mg of naproxen, respectively)	**Analgesia, Dysmenorrhea, Acute Tendonitis and Bursitis:** 1000 mg once daily po. **Acute Gout:** 1000 - 1500 mg once daily po on the first day, followed by 1000 mg once daily until the attack has subsided. **Rheumatoid Arthritis, Osteoarthritis and Ankylosing Spondylitis:** 750 - 1000 mg once daily po.
Netilmicin Sulfate (*)	NETROMYCIN	Antibacterial	Inj: 100 mg/mL	**Urinary Tract Infections (Complicated):** 1.5 - 2.0 mg/kg q 12 h IM or IV. **Serious Systemic Infections:** 1.3 - 2.2 mg/kg q 8 h IM or IV; or, 2.0 - 3.25 mg/kg q 12 h IM or IV.
Nitrofurantoin	FURADANTIN	Urinary Tract Anti-Infective, Antibacterial	Oral Susp: 25 mg/5 mL	50 - 100 mg qid po with food. For long-term suppressive therapy, reduce dosage to 50 - 100 mg po hs.
Nitrofurantoin Macrocrystals	MACRODANTIN	Urinary Tract Anti-Infective, Antibacterial	Cpsl: 25, 50, 100 mg	**Usual Dosage:** 50 - 100 mg qid po with food. **Urinary Tract Infections (Uncomplicated):** 50 mg qid po with food.

GENERIC NAME	COMMON TRADE NAMES	THERAPEUTIC CATEGORY	PREPARATIONS	COMMON ADULT DOSAGE
Ofloxacin (*)	FLOXIN FLOXIN I.V.	Antibacterial	Tab: 200, 300, 400 mg Inj (per mL): 10, 20 mg	**Lower Respiratory Tract, Skin & Skin Structure Infections:** 400 mg q 12 h po or by IV infusion (over 60 min.) for 10 days. **Gonorrhea (Uncomplicated):** 400 mg po or by IV infusion (over 60 min.) as a single dose. **Cervicitis or Urethritis due to *N. gonorrhoeae* and/or *C. trachomatis*:** 300 mg q 12 h po or by IV infusion (over 60 min.) for 7 days. **Acute Pelvic Inflammatory Disease:** 400 mg q 12 h po or by IV infusion (over 60 min.) for 10 - 14 days. **Cystitis due to *E. coli* or *K. pneumoniae*:** 200 mg q 12 h po or by IV infusion (over 60 min.) for 3 days. **Cystitis due to other Organisms:** 200 mg q 12 h po or by IV infusion (over 60 min.) for 7 days. **Urinary Tract Infections (Complicated):** 200 mg q 12 h po or by IV infusion (over 60 min.) for 10 days. **Prostatitis:** 300 mg q 12 h po for 6 weeks or by IV infusion (over 60 min.) for up to 10 days, then switch to oral therapy. (0.5 mL) instilled into the affected ear bid for 14 days.
Orphenadrine Citrate (*)	NORFLEX	Skeletal Muscle Relaxant	Extended-Rel. Tab: 100 mg Inj: 60 mg/2 mL	100 mg bid po, AM and PM. 60 mg q 12 h IM or IV.
Oxacillin Sodium (*)	BACTOCILL	Antibacterial	Cpsl: 250, 500 mg Powd for Inj: 250, 500 mg; 1, 2, 4 g	**Mild to Moderate Infections of the Skin, Soft Tissue or Upper Respiratory Tract:** 500 mg q 4 - 6 h po for a minimum of 5 days. **Serious or Life-Threatening Infections:** After initial parenteral treatment, 1 g q 4 - 6 h po. **Mild to Moderate Upper Respiratory and Local Skin and Soft Tissue Infections:** 250 - 500 mg q 4 - 6 h IM or IV. **Severe Lower Respiratory or Disseminated**

Oxaprozin	DAYPRO	Antiinflammatory	**Tab:** 600 mg	**Infections:** 1 g q 4 - 6 h IM or IV. 1200 mg once daily po. For patients of low body weight or mild disease, an initial dose of 600 mg once a day may be appropriate.
Oxycodone Hydrochloride (*) (C-II)	ROXICODONE	Opioid Analgesic	**Solution:** 5 mg/5 mL **Conc Solution:** 20 mg/mL **Tab:** 5 mg	5 mg q 6 h po prn pain.
	OXYCONTIN		**Controlled-Rel. Tab:** 10, 20, 40, 80 mg	Variable po dosages based on patient tolerance to opioids and type of conversion, e.g., from oral morphine, parenteral morphine, or other opioid analgesics. Commonly used q 12 h.
Oxymorphone Hydrochloride (C-II)	NUMORPHAN	Opioid Analgesic	**Inj (per mL):** 1, 1.5 mg	**IM or SC:** 1 - 1.5 mg q 4 - 6 h, prn pain. **IV:** 0.5 mg q 4 - 6 h, prn pain.
			Rectal Suppos: 5 mg	Insert 1 rectally q 4 - 6 h.
Oxytetracycline (*)	TERRAMYCIN	Antibacterial	**Inj (per mL):** 50, 125 mg	250 mg q 24 h IM or 300 mg daily in divided doses IM at 8- to 12-hour intervals.
Oxytetracycline Hydrochloride (*)	TERRAMYCIN	Antibacterial	**Cpsl:** 250 mg	**Usual Dosage:** 250 - 500 mg q 6 h po. **Brucellosis:** 500 mg qid po with streptomycin for 3 weeks. **Gonorrhea:** Initially 1.5 g po, followed by 500 mg qid po, for a total of 9.0 g. **Syphilis:** 30 - 40 g po in equally divided doses over a period of 10 - 15 days.
Pamidronate Disodium	AREDIA	Bone Stabilizer	**Powd for Inj:** 30, 90 mg	**Hypercalcemia of Malignancy:** **Moderate:** 60 mg - 90 mg by IV infusion (given over ≥ 2 - 24 hours. **Severe:** 90 mg by IV infusion (given over 2 - 24 h. **Paget's Disease:** 30 mg daily by IV infusion (over 4 hours), on 3 consecutive days, for a total dose of 90 mg.

GENERIC NAME	COMMON TRADE NAMES	THERAPEUTIC CATEGORY	PREPARATIONS	COMMON ADULT DOSAGE
Paricalcitol	ZEMPLAR	Vitamin D Analog	Inj: 5 µg/mL	**Osteolytic Bone Lesions of Multiple Myeloma:** 90 mg by IV infusion (over 4 hours) once monthly. Initially 0.04 - 0.1 µg/kg (2.8 - 7 µg) IV (as a bolus injection) no more often than every other day at any time during dialysis. If a satisfactory response is not observed, the dose may be increased by 2 - 4 µg at 2- to 4-week intervals. Doses as high as 0.24 µg/kg (16.8 µg) have been safely given.
Penicillin G Benzathine (*)		Antibacterial	Inj (per mL): 300,000; 600,000 Units	**Streptococcal Upper Respiratory Infections (e.g., Pharyngitis):** 1,200,000 Units IM. **Syphilis (Primary, Secondary & Latent):** 2,400,000 Units IM. **Syphilis (Late):** 2,400,000 Units IM at 7-day intervals for 3 doses. **Rheumatic Fever and Glomerulonephritis (Prophylaxis):** 1,200,000 Units IM once a month or 600,000 Units IM q 2 weeks.
Penicillin G Potassium (*)	PFIZERPEN	Antibacterial	Powd for Inj: 5,000,000; 20,000,000 Units	5,000,000 to 80,000,000 Units daily IM or by IV drip, depending on the severity of the infection and the susceptibility of the infecting organism.
Penicillin G Procaine (*)	PFIZERPEN-AS WYCILLIN	Antibacterial	Inj: 300,000 Units/mL Inj: 600,000 Units/mL	**Usual Dosage:** 600,000 - 1,000,000 Units daily IM. **Syphilis:** 600,000 Units daily IM for 8 - 15 days. **Gonorrhea:** 4,800,000 Units IM divided into at least 2 doses and inj. at diff. sites at the same visit, with probenecid (1 g po).
Penicillin V Potassium (*)	PEN-VEE K	Antibacterial	Tab: 250, 500 mg Powd for Solution (per 5 mL): 125, 250 mg	**Streptococcal Upper Respiratory Infections:** 125 - 250 mg q 6 - 8 h po for 10 days. **Pneumococcal Infections:** 250 - 500 mg q 6 h

po until afebrile for at least 48 hours. **Staphylococcal Infections:** 250 - 500 mg q 6 to 8 h po. **Vincent's Gingivitis and Pharyngitis:** 250 - 500 mg q 6 - 8 h po.

Pentazocine Lactate (*) (C-IV)	TALWIN	Opioid Analgesic	**Inj:** 30 mg/mL	**Usual Dosage:** 30 mg q 3 - 4 h IM, SC or IV. **Patients in Labor:** 30 mg IM or 20 mg q 2 - 3 h IV.
Phytonadione	AQUA-MEPHYTON	Vitamin K$_1$	**Inj (per mL):** 2, 10 mg	2.5 - 25 mg SC or IM. Repeat in 6 - 8 h if necessary.
Piperacillin Sodium (*)	PIPRACIL	Antibacterial	**Powd for Inj:** 2, 3, 4 g	**Urinary Tract Infections (Uncomplicated) and Most Community-Acquired Pneumonia:** 100 to 125 mg/kg/day IM or IV in divided doses q 6 - 12 h. **Urinary Tract Infections (Complicated):** 125 to 200 mg/kg/day IV in divided doses q 6 - 8 h. **Serious Infections:** 200 - 300 mg/kg/day IV in divided doses q 4 - 6 h. **Gonorrhea (Uncomplicated):** 2 g IM as a single dose with probenecid (1 g po).
Piroxicam (*)	FELDENE	Antiinflammatory	**Cpsl:** 10, 20 mg	20 mg daily po.
Prednicarbate	DERMATOP	Corticosteroid	**Cream:** 0.1%	Apply a thin film to skin bid.
Prednisolone	PRELONE	Corticosteroid	**Syrup:** 15 mg/5 mL	Initial dosage varies from 5 - 60 mg daily po depending on the disease being treated and the patient's response.
Prednisolone Acetate	PRED-MILD PRED FORTE	Corticosteroid	**Ophth Susp:** 0.12% **Ophth Susp:** 1%	1 - 2 drops into affected eye(s) bid - qid. During the initial 24 - 48 h, the dosing frequency may be increased if necessary.
Prednisolone Sodium Phosphate	HYDELTRASOL	Corticosteroid	**Inj:** 20 mg/mL	**For IV and IM Injection:** Dose requirements are variable and must be individualized on the basis of the disease and the response of the

GENERIC NAME	COMMON TRADE NAMES	THERAPEUTIC CATEGORY	PREPARATIONS	COMMON ADULT DOSAGE
				patient. The initial dosage varies from 4 to 60 mg a day. Usually the daily parenteral dose of HYDELTRASOL is the same as the oral dose of prednisolone and the dosage interval is q 4 to 8 h. **For Intra-articular, Intralesional and Soft Tissue Injection:** Dose requirements are variable and must be individualized on the basis of the disease, the response of the patient, and the site of injection. The usual dose is from 2 to 30 mg. The frequency usually ranges from once every 3 to 5 days to once every 2 to 3 weeks.
	INFLAMASE MILD 1/8% INFLAMASE FORTE 1%	Corticosteroid	**Opth Solution:** 0.125% **Opth Solution:** 1%	1 - 2 drops into affected eye(s) up to q h during the day & q 2 h at night. When a favorable response occurs, reduce dosage to 1 drop q 4 h.
Prednisone	DELTASONE	Corticosteroid	**Tab:** 2.5, 5, 10, 20, 50 mg	Initial dosage may vary from 5 - 60 mg daily po, depending on the disease being treated.
Propoxyphene Hydrochloride (*) (C-IV)	DARVON	Opioid Analgesic	**Cpsl:** 65 mg	65 mg q 4 h po, prn pain.
Propoxyphene Napsylate (*) (C-IV)	DARVON-N	Opioid Analgesic	**Tab:** 100 mg	100 mg q 4 h po, prn pain.
Risedronate Sodium	ACTONEL	Bone Stabilizer	**Tab:** 5, 30 mg	**Prevention / Treatment of Postmenopausal & Glucocorticoid-Induced Osteoporosis:** 5 mg once daily po. **Paget's Disease:** 30 mg once daily po for 2 months. Take ≥ 30 min. before the first food or drink of the day other than water. Take while in an upright position with a full glass (6 - 8 oz.) of plain water and avoid lying down for 30 min. to minimize the possibility of GI side effects.

Rofecoxib	VIOXX	Antiinflammatory, Non-Opioid Analgesic	Tab: 12.5, 25, 50 mg Susp (per 5 mL): 12.5, 25 mg	**Osteoarthritis:** Initially 12.5 mg once daily po. Some patients may benefit by an increase to the maximum of 25 mg once daily po. **Acute Pain and Primary Dysmenorrhea:** Initially 50 mg once daily po for up to 5 days.
Salsalate	DISALCID	Antiinflammatory	Cpsl: 500 mg Tab: 500, 750 mg	3000 mg daily po, given in divided doses as 1500 mg bid or 1000 mg tid.
SALFLEX			Tab: 500, 750 mg	Same dosage as for DISALCID above.
Silver Sulfadiazine	SSD	Burn Preparation	Cream: 1%	Apply to a thickness of 1/16 inch once or twice daily.
Sulfisoxazole (*)		Antibacterial	Tab: 500 mg	the 1st week, followed by 500 mg bid IM for the 2nd week. **Enterococcal Endocarditis:** 1 g bid IM for 2 weeks, followed by 500 mg bid IM for an additional 4 weeks (with penicillin). Initially 2 - 4 g po, then 4 - 8 g/day divided in 4 - 6 doses.
Sulfisoxazole Acetyl (*)		Antibacterial	Syrup: 500 mg/5 mL (0.9% alcohol)	Initially 2 - 4 g po, then 4 - 8 g/day divided in 4 - 6 doses.
Sulindac (*)	CLINORIL	Antiinflammatory	Tab: 150, 200 mg	**Osteoarthritis, Rheumatoid Arthritis, and Ankyl. Spondylitis:** 150 mg po with food. **Acute Painful Shoulder:** 200 mg bid po with food for 7 - 14 days. **Acute Gouty Arthritis:** 200 mg bid po with food for 7 days.
Tetracycline Hydrochloride (*)	SUMYCIN	Antibacterial	Cpsl & Tab: 250, 500 mg Syrup: 125 mg/5 mL	**Usual Dosage:** 1 - 2 g po divided into 2 or 4 equal doses. **Brucellosis:** 500 mg qid po for 3 weeks with streptomycin. **Syphilis:** 30 - 40 g po in equally divided doses

GENERIC NAME	COMMON TRADE NAMES	THERAPEUTIC CATEGORY	PREPARATIONS	COMMON ADULT DOSAGE
Ticarcillin Disodium (*)	TICAR	Antibacterial	Powd for Inj: 1, 3, 6 g	over a period of 10 - 15 days. **Gonorrhea:** Initially, 1.5 g po followed by 500 mg q 6 h for 4 days (total dose of 9 g). **Uncomplicated Urethral, Endocervical or Rectal Infections due to *Chlamydia trachomatis*:** 500 mg qid po for at least 7 days. **Urinary Tract Infections:** **Uncomplicated:** 1 g IM or direct IV q 6 h. **Complicated:** 150 - 200 mg/kg/day by IV infusion in divided doses q 4 or 6 h. **Most Other Infections:** 200 - 300 mg/kg/day by IV infusion in divided doses q 4 or 6 h.
Ticlopidine Hydrochloride	TICLID	Platelet Aggregation Inhibitor	Tab: 250 mg	250 mg bid po, taken with food.
Tiludronate Sodium	SKELID	Bone Stabilizer	Tab: 240 mg (equivalent to 200 mg of tiludronic acid)	400 mg (acid) po daily with 6 - 8 oz. of water for 3 mos. Do not take within 2 h of food.
Tinzaparin Sodium	INNOHEP	Anticoagulant	Inj: 40000 IUnits/2 mL	175 IU/kg SC once daily for ≥ 6 days and until the patient is adequately anticoagulated with warfarin.
Tizanidine Hydrochloride	ZANAFLEX	Skeletal Muscle Relaxant	Tab: 2, 4 mg	Initially, 4 mg po. May increase by 2 - 4 mg pm q 6 - 8 h to a maximum of 3 doses in 24 h. Maximum: 36 mg per day.
Tobramycin Sulfate (*)	NEBCIN	Antibacterial	Inj (per mL): 10, 40 mg Powd for Inj: 30 mg	**Serious Infections:** 3 mg/kg/day IM or IV in 3 equal doses q 8 h. **Life-Threatening Infections:** Up to 5 mg/kg/day may be given IM or IV in 3 or 4 equal doses.
Tramadol Hydrochloride (*)	ULTRAM	Opioid Analgesic	Tab: 50 mg	50 - 100 mg q 4 - 6 h po, not to exceed 400 mg/day.
Triamcinolone	ARISTOCORT	Corticosteroid	Tab: 1, 2, 4, 8 mg	Initial dose may vary from 4 to 48 mg po per day. Dose requirements are variable and must be individualized based on the disease

333

				and the patient's response.
Triamcinolone Acetonide	KENALOG-10	Corticosteroid	Inj: 10 mg/mL	**Intra-articular or Intrabursal Injection and Injection into Tendon Sheaths**: Initially, 2.5 to 5 mg (for smaller joints) and 5 - 15 mg (for larger joints). **Intradermal Injection**: Varies depending on the disease, but should be limited to 1.0 mg per injection site.
	KENALOG-40		Inj: 40 mg/mL	**IM (deep)**: Usual initial dose is 60 mg. Dosage is usually adjusted from 40 - 80 mg, depending on the patient response and the duration of relief. **Intra-articular or Intrabursal Injection and Injection into Tendon Sheaths**: Initially, 2.5 to 5 mg (for smaller joints) and 5 - 15 mg (for larger joints).
Triamcinolone Diacetate	ARISTOCORT FORTE	Corticosteroid	Inj (per mL): 25, 40 mg	Initial dosage may vary from 3 - 48 mg daily, depending on the specific disease being treated. The average dose is 40 mg IM once a week or 5 - 40 mg intra-articularly or intrasynovially.
Triamcinolone Hexacetonide	ARISTOSPAN	Corticosteroid	Inj (per mL): 5, 20 mg	Initial dosage may vary from 2 - 48 mg daily, depending on the specific disease being treated. The average dose is 2 - 20 mg intra-articularly (depending on the size of the joint), repeated q 3 - 4 weeks. Up to 0.5 mg/square inch of skin may be given by intralesional or sublesional injection.
Trimethoprim (*)	PROLOPRIM	Antibacterial	Tab: 100, 200 mg	100 mg q 12 h po for 10 days, or 200 mg q 24 h po for 10 days.
Trimethoprim Hydrochloride (*)	PRIMSOL	Antibacterial	Solution: 50 mg/5 mL	100 mg bid po for 10 days, or 200 mg once daily po for 10 days.

GENERIC NAME	COMMON TRADE NAMES	THERAPEUTIC CATEGORY	PREPARATIONS	COMMON ADULT DOSAGE
Troleandomycin	TAO	Antibacterial	**Cpsl:** 250 mg	250 - 500 mg qid po.
Trovafloxacin Mesylate (*)	TROVAN	Antibacterial	**Tab:** 100, 200 mg **Inj:** 5 mg/mL (as alatrofloxacin mesylate)	**Community-Acquired Pneumonia and Skin and Skin Structure Infections (Complicated):** 200 mg once daily po or by IV infusion, followed by 200 mg once daily po for 7 - 14 days. **Nosocomial Pneumonia:** 300 mg by IV infusion, followed by 200 mg once daily po for 10 - 14 days. **Gynecologic and Pelvic Infections and Intra-Abdominal Infections (Complicated):** 300 mg by IV infusion, followed by 200 mg once daily po for 7 - 14 days.
Vancomycin Hydrochloride (*)	VANCOCIN HCL	Antibacterial	**Powd for Solution:** 1, 10 g **Cpsl:** 125, 250 mg **Powd for Inj:** 500 mg; 1, 10 g	**Pseudomembranous Colitis:** 500 mg - 2 g daily po in 3 or 4 divided doses for 7 - 10 days. 2 g daily divided either as 500 mg q 6 h or 1 g q 12 h, by IV infusion (at a rate no more than 10 mg/min) over at least 60 minutes.
Warfarin Sodium (*)	COUMADIN	Anticoagulant	**Tab:** 1, 2, 2.5, 3, 4, 5, 6, 7.5, 10 mg **Powd for Inj:** 5 mg	Must be individualized for each patient based on the prothrombin time. Maintenance dosage for most patients is 2 - 10 mg daily po. Individualize dosage. Give as an IV bolus dose over 1 - 2 min into a peripheral vein.

| Zoledronic Acid | ZOMETA | Bone Stabilizer | **Powd for Inj:** 4.264 mg (as the monohydrate equiv. to 4 mg of the anhydrous acid) | **Hypercalcemia of Malignancy:** The maximum recommended dose is 4 mg. This dose must be given as a single dose by IV infusion over ≥ 15 min. Adequately rehydrate the patient prior to drug administration. |

C-II: Controlled Substance, Schedule II
C-III: Controlled Substance, Schedule III
C-IV: Controlled Substance, Schedule IV

SELECTED

COMBINATION

DRUG

PREPARATIONS

C-II: Controlled Substance, Schedule II
C-III: Controlled Substance, Schedule III
C-IV: Controlled Substance, Schedule IV
C-V: Controlled Substance, Schedule V

TRADE NAME	THERAPEUTIC CATEGORY	DOSAGE FORMS AND COMPOSITION	COMMON ADULT DOSAGE
ADVAIR DISKUS	Corticosteroid-Bronchodilator	**Powder for Inhalation:** fluticasone propionate (100 µg), salmeterol (50 µg). **Powder for Inhalation:** fluticasone propionate (250 µg), salmeterol (50 µg). **Powder for Inhalation:** fluticasone propionate (500 µg), salmeterol (50 µg).	1 inhalation bid (approximately 12 h apart). **For the Recommended Starting Strengths, see the Table below.**

For Patients Not Currently on an Inhaled Corticosteroid, it is recommended that the 100 µg / 50 µg strength be used to start.

For Patients Currently on an Inhaled Corticosteroid, the recommended strengths to start with are:

Current Daily Dose of Inhaled Corticosteroid		Recommended Strength of ADVAIR DISKUS
Beclomethasone Dipropionate	≤ 420 µg 462 to 840 µg	100 µg / 50 µg Strength (Use bid.) 250 µg / 50 µg Strength (Use bid.)
Budesonide	≤ 400 µg 800 to 1200 µg 1600 µg	100 µg / 50 µg Strength (Use bid.) 250 µg / 50 µg Strength (Use bid.) 500 µg / 50 µg Strength (Use bid.)
Flunisolide	≤ 1000 µg 1250 to 2000 µg	100 µg / 50 µg Strength (Use bid.) 250 µg / 50 µg Strength (Use bid.)
Fluticasone Propionate Inhalation Aerosol	≤ 176 µg 440 µg 660 to 880 µg	100 µg / 50 µg Strength (Use bid.) 250 µg / 50 µg Strength (Use bid.) 500 µg / 50 µg Strength (Use bid.)
Fluticasone Propionate Inhalation Powder	≤ 200 µg 500 µg 1000 µg	100 µg / 50 µg Strength (Use bid.) 250 µg / 50 µg Strength (Use bid.) 500 µg / 50 µg Strength (Use bid.)

TRADE NAME	THERAPEUTIC CATEGORY	DOSAGE FORMS AND COMPOSITION	COMMON ADULT DOSAGE
AGGRENOX	Platelet Aggregation Inhibitor	**Cpsl:** aspirin (25 mg) [immediate-release], dipyridamole (200 mg) [extended-release]	1 cpsl bid po (1 in the AM and 1 in the PM). Swallow whole; do not chew or crush.
ANALPRAM-HC	Corticosteroid-Local Anesthetic	**Cream:** hydrocortisone acetate (1%), pramoxine HCl (1%). **Cream & Lotion:** hydrocortisone acetate (2.5%), pramoxine HCl (1%)	Apply to the affected area as a thin film tid or qid.

ANEXSIA 5/500 (C-III) ANEXSIA 7.5/650 (C-III) ANEXSIA 10/660 (C-III)	Analgesic	**Tab:** hydrocodone bitatrate (5 mg), acetaminophen (500 mg). **Tab:** hydrocodone bitatrate (7.5 mg), acetaminophen (650 mg). **Tab:** hydrocodone bitatrate (10 mg), acetaminophen (660 mg).	1 - 2 tab q 4 - 6 h po, prn pain. 1 tab q 4 - 6 h po, prn pain. 1 tab q 4 - 6 h po, prn pain.
ARTHROTEC 50	Antiinflammatory	**Enteric-Coated Tab:** diclofenac sodium (50 mg), misoprostol (200 µg).	**Osteoarthritis:** 1 tab tid po. **Rheumatoid Arthritis:** 1 tab tid to qid po.
ARTHROTEC 75	Antiinflammatory	**Enteric-Coated Tab:** diclofenac sodium (75 mg), misoprostol (200 µg).	**Osteoarthritis and Rheumatoid Arthritis:** 1 tab bid po.
AUGMENTIN 125	Antibacterial	**Powd for Susp (per 5 mL):** amoxicillin (125 mg), clavulanic acid (31.25 mg). **Chewable Tab:** amoxicillin (125 mg), clavulanic acid (31.25 mg)	**Usual Dosage:** 1 AUGMENTIN 250 tablet q 8 h po or 1 AUGMENTIN 500 tablet q 12 h po. The 125 mg/5 mL or 250 mg/5 mL suspension may be given in place of the 500 mg tablet.
AUGMENTIN 200		**Powd for Susp (per 5 mL):** amoxicillin (200 mg), clavulanic acid (28.5 mg). **Chewable Tab:** amoxicillin (200 mg), clavulanic acid (28.5 mg)	
AUGMENTIN 250		**Powd for Susp (per 5 mL):** amoxicillin (250 mg), clavulanic acid (62.5 mg). **Chewable Tab:** amoxicillin (250 mg), clavulanic acid (62.5 mg) **Tab:** amoxicillin (250 mg), clavulanic acid (125 mg)	**Severe Infections & Respiratory Infections:** 1 AUGMENTIN 500 tablet q 8 h po or 1 AUGMENTIN 875 tablet q 12 h po. The 200 mg/5 mL or 400 mg/5 mL suspension may be given in place of the 875 mg tablet.
AUGMENTIN 400		**Powd for Susp (per 5 mL):** amoxicillin (400 mg), clavulanic acid (57 mg). **Chewable Tab:** amoxicillin (400 mg), clavulanic acid (57 mg)	
AUGMENTIN 500 AUGMENTIN 875		**Tab:** amoxicillin (500 mg), clavulanic acid (125 mg) **Tab:** amoxicillin (875 mg), clavulanic acid (125 mg)	
BACTRIM	Antibacterial	**Susp (per 5 mL):** sulfamethoxazole (200 mg), trimethoprim (40 mg) **Tab:** sulfamethoxazole (400 mg), trimethoprim (80 mg)	**Urinary Tract Infections:** 1 BACTRIM DS tab, 2 BACTRIM tab or 20 mL of Suspension q 12 h po for 10 - 14 days.

TRADE NAME	THERAPEUTIC CATEGORY	DOSAGE FORMS AND COMPOSITION	COMMON ADULT DOSAGE
BACTRIM DS		Tab: sulfamethoxazole (800 mg), trimethoprim (160 mg)	**Shigellosis:** 1 BACTRIM DS tab, 2 BACTRIM tab or 20 mL of Suspension q 12 h for 5 days. **Acute Exacerbations of Chronic Bronchitis:** 1 BACTRIM DS tab, 2 BACTRIM tab or 20 mL of Suspension q 12 h po for 14 days. *P. carinii* **Pneumonia Treatment:** 20 mg/kg trimethoprim and 100 mg/kg sulfamethoxazole per 24 h in equally divided doses q 6 h for 14 days. *P. carinii* **Pneumonia Prophylax.:** 1 BACTRIM DS tab, 2 BACTRIM tab or 20 mL of Suspension q 24 h po. **Travelers' Diarrhea:** 1 BACTRIM DS tab, 2 BACTRIM tab or 20 mL of Suspension q 12 h po for 5 days.
BACTRIM I.V. INFUSION	Antibacterial	Inj (per 5 mL): sulfamethoxazole (400 mg), trimethoprim (80 mg)	**Severe Urinary Tract Infections and Shigellosis:** 8 - 10 mg/kg daily (based on trimethoprim) in 2 - 4 equally divided doses q 6, 8 or 12 h by IV infusion for up to 14 days for UTI and 5 days for shigellosis. *P. carinii* **Pneumonia:** 15 - 20 mg/kg daily (based on trimethoprim) in 3 - 4 equally divided doses q 6 - 8 h by IV infusion for up to 14 days.
BANCAP HC (C-III)	Analgesic	Cpsl: hydrocodone bitartrate (5 mg), acetaminophen (500 mg)	1 cpsl q 6 h po, prn pain. Maximum: 2 cpsl q 6 h po.

340

BAYER PLUS, EXTRA-STRENGTH	Analgesic	Cplt: aspirin (500 mg), calcium carbonate	1 - 2 cplt q 4 - 6 h po. Max. of 8 cplt in 24 h.
BAYER PM, EXTRA-STRENGTH	Analgesic-Sedative	Cplt: aspirin (500 mg), diphenhydramine HCI (25 mg)	2 cplt hs po.
BICILLIN C-R	Antibacterial	Inj (per mL): penicillin G benzathine (150,000 Units), penicillin G procaine (150,000 Units). Inj (per mL): penicillin G benzathine (300,000 Units), penicillin G procaine (300,000 Units).	**Streptococcal Infections:** 2,400,000 Units by deep IM injection (multiple sites). **Pneumococcal Infections (except Meningitis):** 1,200,000 Units by deep IM injection, repeated q 2 - 3 days until the temperature is normal for 48 hours.
BLEPHAMIDE	Antibacterial-Corticosteroid	Ophth Susp: sulfacetamide sodium (10%), prednisolone acetate (0.2%). Ophth Oint: sulfacetamide sodium (10%), prednisolone acetate (0.2%)	1 drop into affected eye(s) bid to qid. Apply to affected eye(s) tid - qid and once or twice at night.
COLY-MYCIN S OTIC	Antibacterial-Corticosteroid	Otic Susp (per mL): neomycin sulfate (4.71 mg, equivalent to 3.3 mg neomycin base), colistin sulfate (3 mg), hydrocortisone acetate (10 mg = 1%)	5 instilled drops into the affected ear(s) tid - qid.
CORTISPORIN	Antibacterial-Corticosteroid	Ophth Susp (per mL): polymyxin B sulfate (10,000 Units), neomycin sulfate (equal to 3.5 mg of neomycin base), hydrocortisone (10 mg = 1%)	1 - 2 drops into the affected eye(s) q 3 - 4 h, depending on the severity of the condition.
CORTISPORIN OTIC	Antibacterial-Corticosteroid	Otic Solution & Susp (per mL): polymyxin B sulfate (10,000 Units), neomycin sulfate (equal to 3.5 mg of neomycin base), hydrocortisone (10 mg = 1%)	4 drops instilled in the affected ear(s) tid to qid.
DARVOCET-N 50 (C-IV)	Analgesic	Tab: propoxyphene napsylate (50 mg), acetaminophen (325 mg).	2 tab q 4 h prn pain po.
DARVOCET-N 100 (C-IV)		Tab: propoxyphene napsylate (100 mg), acetaminophen (650 mg)	1 tab q 4 h prn pain po.

TRADE NAME	THERAPEUTIC CATEGORY	DOSAGE FORMS AND COMPOSITION	COMMON ADULT DOSAGE
DARVON COMPOUND-65 (C-IV)	Analgesic	**Cpsl:** propoxyphene HCl (65 mg), aspirin (389 mg), caffeine (32.4 mg).	1 cpsl q 4 h po, prn pain.
DECADRON W/XYLOCAINE	Corticosteroid-Local Anesthetic	**Inj (per mL):** dexamethasone sodium phosphate (4 mg), lidocaine HCl (10 mg)	Initial dose ranges from 0.1 to 0.75 mL by injection. Some patients respond to a single injection; in others, additional doses may be needed, usually at 4 - 7 day intervals.
EMPIRIN W/CODEINE #3 (C-III) #4 (C-III)	Analgesic	**Tab:** aspirin (325 mg), codeine phosphate (30 mg) **Tab:** aspirin (325 mg), codeine phosphate (60 mg)	1 - 2 tab q 4 h po, prn. 1 tab q 4 h po, prn.
EXCEDRIN, ASPIRIN FREE	Analgesic	**Cplt & Geltab:** acetaminophen (500 mg), caffeine (65 mg)	2 cplt (or geltabs) q 6 h po while symptoms persist.
EXCEDRIN EXTRA-STRENGTH	Analgesic	**Tab, Cplt & Geltab:** acetaminophen (250 mg), aspirin (250 mg), caffeine (65 mg)	2 tabs (cplt or geltabs) q 6 h po while symptoms persist.
EX-LAX GENTLE STRENGTH	Irritant Laxative-Stool Softener	**Cplt:** sennosides (10 mg), docusate sodium (65 mg)	2 cplts once or twice daily po.
FIORICET	Analgesic	**Tab:** acetaminophen (325 mg), butalbital (50 mg), caffeine (40 mg)	1 - 2 tab q 4 h po. Maximum of 6 tabs daily.
FIORICET W/CODEINE (C-III)	Analgesic	**Cpsl:** acetaminophen (325 mg), butalbital (50 mg), caffeine (40 mg), codeine phosphate (30 mg)	1 - 2 cpsl q 4 h po. Maximum of 6 cpsls daily.
FIORINAL (C-III)	Analgesic	**Cpsl & Tab:** aspirin (325 mg), caffeine (40 mg), butalbital (50 mg)	1 - 2 cpsl (or tab) q 4 h po. Maximum of 6 daily.
FIORINAL W/CODEINE (C-III)	Analgesic	**Cpsl:** aspirin (325 mg), caffeine (40 mg), butalbital (50 mg), codeine phosphate (30 mg)	1 - 2 cpsl q 4 h po. Maximum of 6 cpsls daily.
FML-S	Antibacterial-Corticosteroid	**Ophth Susp:** sulfacetamide sodium (10%), fluorometholone (0.1%)	1 drop in affected eye(s) qid.

342

Drug	Category	Composition	Dosage
HYDROCET (C-III)	Analgesic	**Cpsl:** hydrocodone bitartrate (5 mg), acetaminophen (500 mg)	1 - 2 cpsl q 4 - 6 h po, prn pain.
LORTAB (C-III)	Analgesic	**Elixir (per 5 mL):** hydrocodone bitartrate (2.5 mg), acetaminophen (120 mg), alcohol (7%)	15 mL q 4 h po, prn pain.
LORTAB 2.5/500 (C-III) LORTAB 5/500 (C-III) LORTAB 7.5/500 (C-III) LORTAB 10/500 (C-III)		**Tab:** hydrocodone bitartrate (2.5 mg), acetaminophen (500 mg) **Tab:** hydrocodone bitartrate (5 mg), acetaminophen (500 mg) **Tab:** hydrocodone bitartrate (7.5 mg), acetaminophen (500 mg) **Tab:** hydrocodone bitartrate (10 mg), acetaminophen (500 mg)	1 - 2 tab q 4 - 6 h po, prn pain. 1 - 2 tab q 4 - 6 h po, prn pain. 1 tab q 4 - 6 h po, prn pain. 1 tab q 4 - 6 h po, prn pain.
NORGESIC	Skeletal Muscle Relaxant-Analgesic	**Tab:** orphenadrine citrate (25 mg), aspirin (385 mg), caffeine (30 mg)	1 - 2 tab tid or qid po.
NORGESIC FORTE		**Tab:** orphenadrine citrate (50 mg), aspirin (770 mg), caffeine (60 mg)	1 tab tid or qid po.
PEDIOTIC	Antibacterial-Corticosteroid	**Otic Susp (per mL):** polymyxin B sulfate (10,000 Units), neomycin sulfate (equal to 3.5 mg of neomycin base), hydrocortisone (10 mg = 1%)	4 drops into the affected ear(s) tid to qid
PERCOCET 2.5/325 (C-II) PERCOCET 5/325 (C-II) PERCOCET 7.5/500 (C-II) PERCOCET 10/650 (C-II)	Analgesic	**Tab:** oxycodone HCl (2.5 mg), acetaminophen (325 mg) **Tab:** oxycodone HCl (5 mg), acetaminophen (325 mg) **Tab:** oxycodone HCl (7.5 mg), acetaminophen (500 mg) **Tab:** oxycodone HCl (10 mg), acetaminophen (650 mg)	2 tabs q 6 h po, prn pain. 1 tab q 6 h po, prn pain. 1 tab q 6 h po, prn pain. 1 tab q 6 h po, prn pain.
PERCODAN (C-II)	Analgesic	**Tab:** oxycodone HCl (4.5 mg), oxycodone terephthalate (0.38 mg), aspirin (325 mg)	1 tab q 6 h po, prn pain.
PERCODAN-DEMI (C-II)	Analgesic	**Tab:** oxycodone HCl (2.25 mg), oxycodone terephthalate (0.19 mg), aspirin (325 mg)	1 - 2 tab q 6 h po, prn pain.
PERCOGESIC	Analgesic-Antihistamine	**Cplt:** acetaminophen (325 mg), phenyltoloxamine citrate (30 mg)	2 cplt q 6 h po.
PERCOGESIC EXTRA-STRENGTH	Analgesic-Antihistamine	**Cplt:** acetaminophen (500 mg), diphenhydramine HCl (12.5 mg)	2 cplt q 6 h po.
PERI-COLACE	Irritant Laxative-Stool Softener	**Cpsl:** casanthranol (30 mg), docusate sodium (100 mg) **Syrup (per 15 mL):** casanthranol (30 mg), docusate sodium (60 mg), alcohol (10%)	1 - 2 cpsls hs po. 15 - 30 mL hs po.

343

TRADE NAME	THERAPEUTIC CATEGORY	DOSAGE FORMS AND COMPOSITION	COMMON ADULT DOSAGE
PHRENILIN PHRENILIN FORTE	Analgesic	**Tab:** acetaminophen (325 mg), butalbital (50 mg). **Cpsl:** acetaminophen (650 mg), butalbital (50 mg).	1 - 2 tab q 4 h po, prn. 1 cpsl q 4 h po, prn.
POLY-PRED	Antibacterial-Corticosteroid	**Ophth Suspension (per mL):** neomycin sulfate (equal to 3.5 mg of neomycin base), polymyxin B sulfate (10,000 Units), prednisolone acetate (0.5%)	1 or 2 drops q 3 - 4 h into affected eye(s). Acute infections may require dosing q 30 minutes, initially.
PRED-G	Antibacterial-Corticosteroid	**Ophth Suspension:** gentamicin sulfate (0.3%), prednisolone acetate (1.0%)	1 drop into affected eye(s) bid to qid. During the initial 24 to 48 h, dosage may be raised
PRIMAXIN I.M.	Antibacterial	**Powd for Inj:** imipenem (500 mg), cilastatin sodium (500 mg) **Powd for Inj:** imipenem (750 mg), cilastatin sodium (750 mg)	**Lower Respiratory Tract, Skin & Skin Structure, and Gynecologic Infections:** 500 or 750 mg (of imipenem) q 12 h IM. **Intra-Abdominal Infections:** 750
PRIMAXIN I.V.	Antibacterial	**Powd for Inj:** imipenem (250 mg), cilastatin sodium (250 mg) **Powd for Inj:** imipenem (500 mg), cilastatin sodium (500 mg)	Administer by IV infusion. Each 250 or 500 mg dose (of imipenem) should be given over 20 - 30 min. Each 1000 mg dose should be infused over 40 - 60 min. **Infections:** **Mild:** 250 - 500 mg q 6 h. **Moderate:** 500 - 1000 mg q 6 to 8 h. **Severe, Life-Threatening:** 500 mg q 6 h to 1000 mg q 6 to 8 h. **Urinary Tract (Uncomplicated):** 250 mg q 6 h. **Urinary Tract (Complicated):** 500 mg q 6 h.
PROCTOCREAM-HC	Local Anesthetic-Corticosteroid	**Cream:** pramoxine HCl (1%), hydrocortisone acetate (1%)	Apply to the affected area as a thin film tid - qid.

PROCTOFOAM-HC	Local Anesthetic-Corticosteroid	**Aerosol:** pramoxine HCl (1%), hydrocortisone acetate (1%)	Apply to the affected area tid to qid.
ROBAXISAL	Skeletal Muscle Relaxant-Analgesic	**Tab:** methocarbamol (400 mg), aspirin (325 mg)	2 tab qid po. 3 tab qid po may be used in severe conditions for 1 - 3 days in patients who are able to tolerate salicylates.
ROXICET	Analgesic	**Tab:** oxycodone HCl (5 mg), acetaminophen (325 mg) **Solution (per 5 mL):** oxycodone HCl (5 mg), acetaminophen (325 mg), alcohol (0.4%)	1 tab q 6 h po, prn pain. 5 mL q 6 h po, prn pain.
ROXICET 5/500	Analgesic	**Cplt:** oxycodone HCl (5 mg), acetaminophen (500 mg)	1 cplt q 6 h po, prn pain.
ROXILOX	Analgesic	**Cpsl:** oxycodone HCl (5 mg), acetaminophen (500 mg)	1 cpsl q 6 h po, prn pain.
ROXIPRIN	Analgesic	**Tab:** oxycodone HCl (4.5 mg), oxycodone terephthalate (0.38 mg), aspirin (325 mg)	1 tab q 6 h po, prn pain.
SEPTRA	Antibacterial	**Susp (per 5 mL):** sulfamethoxazole (200 mg), trimethoprim (40 mg) **Tab:** sulfamethoxazole (400 mg), trimethoprim (80 mg)	**Urinary Tract Infections:** 1 SEPTRA DS tab, 2 SEPTRA tab or 20 mL of Suspension q 12 h po for 10 - 14 days. **Shigellosis:** 1 SEPTRA DS tab, 2 SEPTRA tab or 20 mL of Suspension for 5 days.
SEPTRA DS		**Tab:** sulfamethoxazole (800 mg), trimethoprim (160 mg)	**Acute Exacerbations of Chronic Bronchitis:** 1 SEPTRA DS tab, 2 SEPTRA tab or 20 mL of Susp. q 12 h po for 14 days. **P. carinii Pneumonia Treatment:** 20 mg/kg trimethoprim and 100 mg/kg sulfamethoxazole per 24 h in equally divided doses q 6 h for 14 days. **P. carinii Pneumonia Prophylax.:** 1 SEPTRA DS tab, 2 SEPTRA tab or 20 mL of Suspension q 24 h po.

345

TRADE NAME	THERAPEUTIC CATEGORY	DOSAGE FORMS AND COMPOSITION	COMMON ADULT DOSAGE
			Travelers' Diarrhea: 1 SEPTRA DS tab, 2 SEPTRA tab or 20 mL of Suspension q 12 h po for 5 days.
SEPTRA I.V. INFUSION	Antibacterial	Inj **(per 5 mL):** sulfamethoxazole (400 mg), trimethoprim (80 mg)	**Severe Urinary Tract Infections and Shigellosis:** 8 - 10 mg/kg daily (based on trimethoprim) in 2 - 4 equally divided doses q 6, 8 or 12 h by IV infusion for up to 14 days for UTI and 5 days for shigellosis. **P. carinii Pneumonia:** 15 - 20 mg/kg daily (based on trimethoprim) in 3 - 4 equally divided doses q 6 - 8 h by IV infusion for up to 14 days.
SOMA COMPOUND	Skeletal Muscle Relaxant-Analgesic	**Tab:** carisoprodol (200 mg), aspirin (325 mg)	1 - 2 tab qid po.
SOMA COMPOUND W/ CODEINE (C-III)	Skeletal Muscle Relaxant-Analgesic	**Tab:** carisoprodol (200 mg), aspirin (325 mg), codeine phosphate (16 mg)	1 - 2 tab qid po.
SYNERCID	Antibacterial	**Powd for Inj:** quinupristin (150 mg), dalfopristin (350 mg)	**Vancomycin-resistant *E. faecium* Bacteremia:** 7.5 mg/kg q 8 h by IV infusion (over 60 min.). Duration of therapy dependent on site of infection and severity. **Complicated Skin and Skin-Structure Infections:** 7.5 mg/kg q 12 h by IV infusion (over 60 min.) for at least 7 days.
TALACEN (C-IV)	Analgesic	**Tab:** pentazocine HCl (equal to 25 mg pentazocine base), acetaminophen (650 mg)	1 tab q 4 h po, prn pain.

TALWIN COMPOUND (C-IV)	Analgesic	Cplt: pentazocine HCl (equal to 12.5 mg pentazocine base), aspirin (325 mg)	2 cplt tid or qid po, prn pain.
TALWIN NX	Analgesic	Tab: pentazocine HCl (equal to 50 mg pentazocine base), naloxone HCl (0.5 mg)	1 tab q 3 - 4 h po.
TRILISATE	Non-Opioid Analgesic, Antipyretic, Antiinflammatory	Tab: choline magnesium salicylate (500 mg as: choline salicylate (293 mg) and magnesium salicylate (362 mg)) Tab: choline magnesium salicylate (750 mg as: choline salicylate (440 mg) and magnesium salicylate (544 mg)) Tab: choline magnesium salicylate (1000 mg as: choline salicylate (587 mg) and magnesium salicylate (725 mg)) Liquid (per 5 mL): choline magnesium salicylate (500 mg as: choline salicylate (293 mg) and magnesium salicylate (362 mg))	**Pain & Fever:** 1000 - 1500 mg bid po. **Inflammation:** 1500 mg bid po or 3000 mg once daily hs po.
TYLENOL W/CODEINE (C-V)	Analgesic	Elixir (per 5 mL): acetaminophen (120 mg), codeine phosphate (12 mg), alcohol (7%)	15 mL q 4 h po, prn pain.
TYLENOL W/CODEINE #2 (C-III) #3 (C-III) #4 (C-III)	Analgesic	Tab: acetaminophen (300 mg), codeine phosphate (15 mg). Tab: acetaminophen (300 mg), codeine phosphate (30 mg). Tab: acetaminophen (300 mg), codeine phosphate (60 mg).	2 - 3 tab q 4 h po, prn pain. 1 - 2 tab q 4 h po, prn pain. 1 tab q 4 h po, prn pain.
TYLOX (C-II)	Analgesic	Cpsl: oxycodone HCl (5 mg), acetaminophen (500 mg)	1 cpsl q 6 h po, prn pain.
ULTRACET	Analgesic	Tab: tramadol HCl (37.5 mg), acetaminophen (325 mg)	2 tabs q 4 - 6 h po.
UNASYN	Antibacterial	Powd for Inj: 1.5 g (1 g ampicillin sodium, 0.5 g sulbactam sodium) Powd for Inj: 3.0 g (2 g ampicillin sodium, 1 g sulbactam sodium)	1.5 - 3.0 g q 6 h by deep IM inj, by slow IV injection (over at least 10 - 15 min), or by IV infusion (diluted with 50 - 100 mL of a compatible diluent and given over 15 - 30 mins).
VASOCIDIN	Antibacterial-Corticosteroid	Ophth Solution: sulfacetamide sodium (10%), prednisolone acetate (0.25%)	2 drops into affected eye(s) q 4 h. Prolong dosing interval as

347

TRADE NAME	THERAPEUTIC CATEGORY	DOSAGE FORMS AND COMPOSITION	COMMON ADULT DOSAGE
		Ophth Oint: sulfacetamide sodium (10%), prednisolone acetate (0.5%)	the condition improves. Apply to affected eye(s) tid or qid during the day and 1 - 2 times at night.
VICODIN (C-III) VICODIN ES (C-III)	Analgesic	**Tab:** hydrocodone bitartrate (5 mg), acetaminophen (500 mg) **Tab:** hydrocodone bitartrate (7.5 mg), acetaminophen (750 mg)	1 - 2 tab q 4 - 6 h po, prn pain. 1 tab q 4 - 6 h po, prn pain.
VICODIN HP		**Tab:** hydrocodone bitartrate (10 mg), acetaminophen (660 mg)	1 tab q 4 - 6 h po, prn pain.
VICOPROFEN	Analgesic	**Tab:** hydrocodone bitartrate (7.5 mg), ibuprofen (200 mg)	1 tab q 4 - 6 h po, prn pain.
WYGESIC (C-IV)	Analgesic	**Tab:** propoxyphene HCl (65 mg), acetaminophen (650 mg)	1 tab q 4 h po, prn pain.
ZOSYN	Antibacterial	**Powd for Inj:** 2.25 g (2 g piperacillin, 0.25 g tazobactam) **Powd for Inj:** 3.375 g (3 g piperacillin, 0.375 g tazobactam) **Powd for Inj:** 4.5 g (4 g piperacillin, 0.5 g tazobactam)	**Usual Dosage:** 12 g/1.5 g daily by IV infusion (over 30 min), given as 3.375 g q 6 h. **Nosocomial Pneumonia:** 3.375 g q 4 h by IV infusion (over 30 min) plus an aminoglycoside.
ZYDONE (C-III)	Analgesic	**Cpsl:** hydrocodone bitartrate (5 mg), acetaminophen (500 mg)	1 - 2 cpsl q 4 - 6 h po, prn pain.

C-II: Controlled Substance, Schedule II
C-III: Controlled Substance, Schedule III
C-IV: Controlled Substance, Schedule IV
C-V: Controlled Substance, Schedule V

INDEX

INDEX

INDEX

INDEX

INDEX

INDEX

INDEX

INDEX

INDEX

INDEX

INDEX

ORDER FORM

PHONE	FAX	VIA WEB SITE
1-800-417-3189	1-215-657-1475	MEDICALSURVEILLANCE.COM

E-MAIL	CHECKS OR MONEY ORDERS	MAIL
MEDSURVEILLANCE@AOL.COM	Make check payable to MSI and mail order form	P.O. Box 480 Willow Grove, Pa. 19090

Books	Price	Qty	Sub-Total
Handbook of Commonly Prescribed Drugs with Therapeutic, Toxic and Lethal Levels, 18th Edition (2003) ISBN # 0-942447-44-1	$ 25.50		
Handbook of Common Orthopaedic Fractures and Drugs, 1st Edition (2003) ISBN # 0-942447-43-3	$ 19.95		
Travelers Guide to International Drugs, **Western Hemisphere** (2001) ISBN # 942447-40-9	$ 14.00		
Travelers Guide to International Drugs, **European Volume I ** (2001) ISBN # 942447-39-5	$ 14.00		
Travelers Guide to International Drugs, **European Volume II ** (2001) ISBN # 942447-38-7	$ 14.00		
Travelers Guide to International Drugs, **Middle & Far East** (2001) ISBN # 0-942447-32-8	$ 14.00		
Handbook of Commonly Prescribed Pediatric Drugs, 6th Edition (1999) ISBN # 0-942447-27-1	$ 18.50		
Antimicrobial Therapy in Primary Care Medicine, 1st Edition (1997) ISBN # 0-942447-22-0	$ 17.00		
Drug Charts in Basic Pharmacology, 3rd Edition (2000) ISBN # 0-942447-37-9	$ 18.95		
Warning: Drugs in Sports, 1st Edition (1995) ISBN # 0-942447-16-6	$ 14.50		

Shipping and Handling Charges:			
Add $ 6.50 for orders between $10.00 - $49.99	SUB-TOTAL		
Add $ 9.00 for orders between $50.00 - $ 99.99	(*) Shipping & Handling		
Add $ 11.00 for orders between $100.00 - 149.99	PA Residents, Add 6% Sales Tax		
Add $ 13.00 for orders Greater then $ 150.00	TOTAL		

Bookstores subject to standard shipping and handling charges

Name: _____

Address: _____

City: _____ STATE: _____ ZIP: _____

E-Mail Address: _____

AMT. ENCLOSED _____ ☐ VISA ☐ M/C ☐ DISCOVER ☐ AMERICAN EXPRESS ☐ CHECK

CARD NUMBER: _____ EXP. DATE: _____

AUTHORIZED SIGNATURE _____ PHONE: _____

If you are paying by credit card, Call Toll Free or Fax

REQUEST FOR INFORMATION

If you wish to be placed on a mailing list for information concerning new publications and updates, please fill out the form below and mail to:

MEDICAL SURVEILLANCE INC.
P.O. Box 480   Willow Grove, PA 19090

(PLEASE PRINT)

Name

Organization

Street Address

City_____State

Zip Code

Telephone Number (Optional)

FOR FURTHER INFORMATION CALL:
800 - 417-3189 or 215 - 784-0976

E-Mail us at **medsurveillance@aol.com**

Visit Us on the **World Wide Web** at
hhtp://www.medicalsurveillance.com